AfricaPraying

A Handbook on HIV/AIDS Sensitive Sermon Guidelines and Liturgy

Edited by: Musa W.Dube

Contributing Writers:
*Isabel Apawo Phiri *Ezra Chitando *Tinyiko S. Maluleke
*Felicidade Chirenda *Canon Gideon Byamugisha
*Gladies Jeco *Prince Moiseraela Dibeela* Fulata L. Moyo
*Musa W. Dube *Augustine C. Musopole *Cheryl Dibeela

The first printing of this book was produced
for the eighth general assembly of the
All Africa Conference of Churches,
22 to 27 November 2003, Yaoundé, Cameroon.

ISBN 2-8254-1407-7

2003
Second Printing 2004
Third Printing November 2004

World Council of Churches
150 route de Ferney, P.O. Box 2100
1211 Geneva 2
Switzerland

Website: http://www.wcc-coe.org

Table of Contents

Notes on Contributors

Commissioner Revd. Canon Gideon Byamugisha is an Anglican priest from Uganda. He is currently serving under World Vision International as Church/FBO Partnership Advisor, HIV/AIDS Hope Initiative. His e-mail Address: gideon_Byamugisha@wvi.org

Rev. Felicidade Cherinda is an ordained Presbyterian minister from Mozambique. She is currently serving in a Minister in Maputo. Her e-mail is: cherinda@teledata.mz

Dr Ezra Chitando is a member of the Seventh Day Adventists and is from Zimbabwe. He is currently serving as lecturer of World Religions and Dean of student affairs at the University of Zimbabwe. His e-mail is: chitsa21@yahoo.com

Revd. Cheryl Dibeela is an ordained minister of the United Congregational Church of Southern Africa, and is from Botswana. Currently she is running Mabogo Dinku, a community development project, as coordinator and founder. Her e-mail is: cherylnatalie@yahoo.com

Revd. Moiseraele P. Dibeela is an ordained minister of the United Congregational Church of Southern Africa, and is from Botswana. Currently he is the principal of Kgolagano Theological College. His e-mail is: kgolagano@mega.bw

Professor Musa W. Dube is member of United Methodist Church, and is from Botswana. She holds a teaching post at the University of Botswana as a New Testament lecturer. Currently she is serving as an HIV/AIDS and theological consultant for churches in Africa under the World Council of Churches. Her e-mail is: wenkosi@hotmail.com

Revd. Gladies Jeco is an ordained minister of the Presbyterian Church, and is from Mozambique. She is currently serving a congregation at Ricatla Theological College.

Professor Tinyiko S. Maluleke is an ordained minister of the Presbyterian Church, and is from South Africa. He is professor of black theology. Currently he is serving as the Dean of the faculty of theology in UNISA, Pretoria. His e-mail is: malults@unisa.ac.za.

Ms. Fulata L. Moyo is a Presbyterian from Malawi. Currently she is a lecturer at Chancellor College, University of Malawi. Her e-mail is: fulamoyo@yahoo.com

Revd. Dr Agustine C. Musopole is an ordained minister of the Church of Central Africa, and is from Malawi. Currently he is serving as the Secretary General of the Malawi Council of Churches. His e- mail address is: mipingo@malawi.net

Professor Isabel Phiri is the Coordinator of the Circle of Concerned African Women Theologians, and the Director of the Center for Constructive Theology, and Professor of African Theology at the school of Theology, University of Natal. She is a Scottsville Presbyterian, and is from Malawi, though she is currently living in South Africa. Her e-mail is: Phiri1@nu.ac.za

Introduction: AfricaPraying

HIV/AIDS Challenges and the Church

Since the outbreak of HIV/AIDS, the average church leader's work in the African continent has doubled; there are more sick people who need to be visited and prayed for; there are more grieved relatives who need to be visited and encouraged; and there are an increasing number of orphans who cannot be absorbed by their overburdened extended families and who need to be comforted, cared for, guided, loved and put in day care-centers. There are more desperate widows who are grieved and who may be impoverished by the sickness of their former husbands or dispossessed by relatives, and who need counseling care and support. There are more grandparents grieved by the death of their children and burdened by care for their orphaned grand children. There are many who are dying and need to be prepared to die peacefully and with dignity; and there are many who are dead, who must be buried. There are millions of people living with HIV/AIDS (PLWHAs) who are confronting enormous stigma, and who need counseling. Whole communities are lost in hopelessness, despair and fear, and must be brought to see and know God's unfailing presence even at this tragic time. Lastly, there are the majority, who are not infected and who must be helped to stay safe.

One can go on outlining. The work is enormous. Of course, there are many other HIV/AIDS players; the governments, NGOs and the private sector all doing their parts in restoring healing to a broken people. Yet the church and its leaders, by virtue of their community centeredness, their close relationship with individuals and families, their value of holding each person as God's person, and their role as servants of God, bearers of salvation and hope, have much expected from them. Much is laid at the feet of the church in the HIV/AIDS struggle. The challenge is in confronting the African church.

Obviously, this does not mean that the average church leader (and the church members) automatically have the skills or are well equipped to deal with HIV/AIDS, for this is a relatively new epidemic. Most ministers who are serving now, never learned about HIV/AIDS in their theological training programs. They were not instructed on HIV/AIDS counseling, prevention and care, or HIV/AIDS project/program design and management, and yet they are expected to stand up to the challenge. Many church ministers were not instructed in reading the Bible from the HIV/AIDS context. They were not instructed on preaching in an HIV/AIDS context. They do not have liturgy that specifically addresses HIV/AIDS. How should the church and its leaders deal with prevention, and the origin and meaning of HIV/AIDS? How should they deal with the HIV/AIDS stigma? How should they address the needs of the affected: orphans, widows, grandparents, grieved relatives, dying people and hopeless communities? How should they minister to the infected who are living with HIV/AIDS and facing enormous stigma? All these questions confront the church leader and worker in the field, often with no ready answers or resources with which to address them. In short, an average church minister is challenged to learn a whole new way of doing ministry in an HIV/AIDS context. The irony, however, is that with the doubled amount of work, there is really no time for any meaningful research, studying or creative space for most church workers. Of course, there is a huge amount of literature produced by governments, NGOs and the private sector on HIV/AIDS. Yet this literature does not necessarily mainstream HIV/AIDS in religion or explore how religion can use its sources in the HIV/AIDS struggle. This task remains to be carried out by the religious institutions themselves: the worship centers and the academic departments of religion, Bible schools and other church related institutions.

In addition to the newness of the epidemic and the enormous amount of work demanded from the church and its leaders, there is a problem of language—the language to address issues of human sexuality. It is not in the practice of the church or of most African cultures to discuss issues of human sexuality openly. In most African cultures, discussions on sexuality were designated to specific spaces, times and individuals. In Southern Africa, for example, this teaching was passed on during initiation schools, when young women and men were being trained on the roles and responsibilities of being adult citizens. The colonial Christian mission was quite deliberate in eliminating these spaces, but tragically, did not make any particular replacement within the church or school programs. Sex education was left to individual families—who were not culturally equipped to do it. In the end, sexual education is not addressed in any formal space. Young people pick ideas from their friends and the media. The church with its own Christian culture of silence demonizes sex, and was obviously not helped by the African cultural context to speak openly about HIV/AIDS.

Lastly, the fact that HIV/AIDS is an epidemic within other social diseases of poverty; gender inequalities; violence; human rights abuse; child abuse; ethnic conflicts/cleansing; national and international injustice; and discrimination on the basis of sexuality, race, age and physical ability; calls for a church whose approach is socially, economically, culturally and politically well informed. The church needs to be socially informed. Its liturgy needs to insist on, and celebrate justice. HIV/AIDS is more than just an individual's lack of morality. Stopping the epidemic will take more than just individual behavior change. There must be a change in the morality of both the individual, as well as the social institutions that people dwell in. Here perhaps, the church leaders are confronted by one of their greatest challenges; for many insist that HIV/AIDS will be eradicated through abstinence and faithfulness (and consequently the infected could be seen as those who are paying for their own failure).

While abstinence and faithfulness are no doubt effective moral values which must continue to be encouraged, the church has been forcefully brought face to face with the fact that individuals are not islands. Real people live within particular economic, cultural, political, and social institutions and structures that determine the decisions they make and implement. Consequently, even when people know and wish to abstain in order to protect themselves from HIV/AIDS, when confronted with hunger, they may choose to get involved in sex work to raise money for food. Even if some women wish to abstain from unfaithful partners, they have to think about loosing shelter and support in cultures that still remain patriarchal—that is cultures in which property and leadership are largely in the hands on men. Even if women are faithful, in cultures where unfaithfulness is culturally tolerated from men, they will still be at risk of infection. Also, families are separated over a long time by labor immigration, displacement of people, through political and economic oppression, and many raging wars, thus making faithfulness in marriage into an unpractical ideal. Further, in war torn zones, abstinence will not protect women from rape, which is used by warring factions to get back at each other. Family, health and education systems do not work in war zones. But worse, rape is no longer confined to war zones, and is on the rise due to myths surrounding HIV/AIDS. With the loss of control that characterizes the HIV/AIDS atmosphere, rape has become a symptom of men's desperate search for control over women's bodies. Young girls, children and infants are raped in their homes, in the streets, by both strangers and their own relatives. Within such a social context, how does it help for church leaders to harp on abstinence and faithfulness as the key to HIV/AIDS prevention? Clearly, we also need to address the social diseases and injustices that promote the spread of HIV/AIDS. We need to seek the healing of all our relationships: our relationships to one another; our relationship with God, and our relationship with the environment. If these relationships are sick, then we are creating an unhealthy world for ourselves and our neighbors—one that is bound to affect us.

The Goal, Contents, and Structure of the Handbook

In the face of the challenges confronting the church and it leaders, a group of writers under the support and leadership of the Ecumenical HIV/AIDS Initiative, sought to produce a resource book for the church and its leaders (minister/pastor, Sunday school teacher, Bible study leader, youth leader, women's and men's fellowships, and the laity). The resource book, *AfricaPraying: A Handbook on HIV/AIDS Sensitive Sermons and Liturgy,* has been produced to assist the church and its leaders to realize their full potential in the HIV/AIDS struggle.

This handbook seeks to equip the church leader/worker with strategies to break the silence and stigma surrounding HIV/AIDS; creating a compassionate and healing church. The handbook seeks also to provide church leaders/workers with tools that will release the full spiritual power, vision, and values of the Christian faith, and enable the church to fight HIV/AIDS. It seeks to help the church leader/workers by underlining how the Christian faith calls us to serve and to heal God's world and people; healing bodies, relationships, institutions and structures, and our relationship with God. Given the newness of the epidemic and the overburdened church leader/worker, this handbook seeks to provide an accessible and user-friendly resource that could be readily used by church leaders/workers to break the silence and stigma, and to call the church to HIV/AIDS prevention, provision of quality care, and mitigation of the impact. If well used, the church leaders/workers will not have to suffer from burn out and stress, given that the struggle against HIV/AIDS will be fully owned by all members of the church, thus raising a strong and formidable army.

The contents of the handbook are comprehensive sermon guidelines that take the HIV/AIDS context into consideration and show how Christian scripture can be a source of transforming energy. The sermon guidelines seek to highlight how the gospel can inform the HIV/AIDS struggle, and activate the church into a body of transformative healers and justice seekers. In this way, the sermon guidelines seek to equip the church to break the silence, to break the stigma, and to awake and energize the church to be a formidable army in the struggle against HIV/AIDS. The structure of the sermon guidelines[1], therefore methodologically seeks to assist the preacher/Bible study/worship leader to walk the audience through a process of: learning, confessing, being thankful, praying, re-envisioning and undertaking concrete plans on what the church can do to change the HIV/AIDS situation. The structure of the sermon guidelines, seeks to assist the preacher in delivering a sermon that will enable the audience translate the ideals of its Christian

---

[1] We are highly indebted to the structural arrangement of Matthias Krieser, *Preacher's Helper: Sermon Preparation for Lutheran Lay Preachers,* Kanye: LUCSA, 2000, which we employed and creatively adapted.

faith into liberating and healing action. They seek to help the church leader/worker to move members and society from numbness of the tragic strike of HIV/AIDS, to an active army of healers, servants of justice and bearers of hope. The introduction of each sermon guideline provides the context of HIV/AIDS for the preacher/Bible study/Sunday School/worship leader. The details of the given text are highlighted for them; the methodological structure is then given; songs, prayers and symbols are provided for the church leader to use as needed.

Despite this provision, the church of Africa is undeniably as diverse as its cultures, contexts and countries. A simplified approach categorizes the church into four groups: mainline, Orthodox/Coptic, African Independent and Evangelical/charismatic churches. Each of these four groups consists of many different traditions in itself. It is therefore, up to each church leader to *re-appropriate and re-interpret* these sermons according to their denomination, context, audience, needs and goals. If one feels comfortable using them as they are written, that is fine, but generally as an ecumenical resource document, this text's completeness lies in the hands of each user within their particular context. To each user I say: "This handbook is yours, to use as your own creative pad, to take whatever you find useful, and take it to new and different levels for your particular context and audience."

I must add that these are not just sermon guidelines, they are also full worship orders. Most include: opening prayers; songs; introductions which highlight the HIV/AIDS context; details of the text; an outline of how the sermon can be applied to individual listeners, congregations, and the larger society; a closing song and prayer; and an outline of various symbols that can be used. Every preacher or worship leader is free to take these guidelines as they are given, to transform them, or to use other alternatives. In particular, in the area of songs and symbols of worship, one cannot assume that the songs chosen by the writers will be known to every Christian church. Nonetheless, we included even new songs. Every user is free to choose appropriate songs; to sing the given songs according to their own created tune; to chant them in a poetry style; or to have young people perform them in a rap style. Moreover, given the orality of the African context, there is a large body of popular choruses, for which we have no idea of the composer. We have acknowledged these songs as community/anonymous/popular songs. But we apologize in advance to those who know themselves as the rightful composers and who wish to be acknowledged.

The area of symbols and objects of worship was equally complicated. The generally accepted Christian symbols of worship are: oil, bread, wine, water, candles, clothes and sound. Even these are used in various ways and have various degrees of acceptability in different traditions. Since the word has dwelt among us, and since the whole creation is God's created world, we were not at all limited to the traditional Christian symbols. Many other symbols of worship can be employed and we outline them. The user is free to utilize symbols from their own context. Yet here again each user will have to judge their own context and audience, and adapt accordingly. However, we also sought to capture the participatory, communal, dramatic and oral spirit of spontaneity that characterizes the worship space of the African church. This was a challenge, for the letter kills the spirit. We believe the worshipping African church will act as a whirlwind for the Holy Spirit; our pens could never come close to such an articulation. Let those who have ears hear, and those who have eyes see!

Coming to the structural presentation of the handbook, it is divided into five parts.
The first section features sermon guideline on life markers. This section seeks to provide

the service leader with resources for mainstreaming HIV/AIDS in celebration services. The second part focuses on church calendar events. The third part of the handbook contains HIV/AIDS sensitive sermons guidelines and liturgy on various themes for general church services, Sunday school classes or Bible study groups. It provides ready resources and methods on how to mainstream HIV/AIDS by addressing themes that are particularly highlighted by the epidemic; such as life, hope, compassion, repentance, healing, forgiveness, love, sexuality, fear, stigma and discrimination, reconciliation, and healing. Thus it features HIV/AIDS sensitive sermon guidelines that focus on children, the boy child, the girl child, youth, parents, single parents, men, grandparents, widows, PLHWHAs, HIV/AIDS workers and activists, homosexuals, and community leaders/workers. This is the longest section, and rightly so, for unless each person and group is addressed and fully equipped, we cannot expect to win the war against HIV/AIDS. Part five focuses on social factors contributing to HIV/AIDS. It seeks to help the church and its leaders to be able to deal with the social epidemics that sponsor HIV/AIDS; namely, poverty and economic injustice, gender inequality, violence of various types, race and ethnic-based discrimination, age based discrimination (children and elders), national and international injustice. While the whole of this book inevitably brings justice and liturgy to a meeting point, it is more specific in this last section.

Obviously, this handbook does not seek to replace the liturgies that various church traditions employ. It seeks to assist every church leader to mainstream HIV/AIDS within their given context, audience and Christian background, so as to build a church that knows and successfully carries out its mission of healing, compassion, hope and justice building. The sermon guidelines of this handbook can, therefore, be used side by side with one's own church liturgies and preaching calendars. They can creatively inform one's own church preaching calendar, Sunday school lessons, women's, men's, and youth services and programs. Be that as it may, I must not fail to say to you, the church of Africa, "*Blessed are those who will decide to use this handbook more consistently, even daring to put aside their formal preaching calendars, for HIV/AIDS matters cannot wait—they are urgent*". They are about saving life from death, despair and hopelessness. They are about healing a hurting and suffering people. A godly and a Christ-like church cannot afford to put these urgent issues of life and death at the periphery. The church must act and act now--we cannot just continue with business as usual, as if HIV/AIDS is not infecting and affecting our congregations and families; recklessly planting hopelessness and despair in our spirits and communities. Let those who have ears hear and act.

The Process of Producing the Handbook

Over the past nine months, a group of writers from different countries and churches have been prayerfully and creatively writing HIV/AIDS sensitive sermons and liturgy for the English and Portuguese speaking African churches and leaders (another group has been working on a French equivalent). Each writer had a maximum of ten passages. In January 2003, soon after the New Year, we met in Mmokolodi Nature Reserve, just outside Gaborone in Botswana, to share what we had been writing, to agree on a working structure, and then we dispersed to re-write again. Both the place and time were deliberately chosen. Botswana, with the highest infection rate in the world, was a good place to gather around the theme of putting up HIV/AIDS sensitive sermon guidelines and liturgy. Second, the nature reserve setting enabled undivided concentration as we reflected on the church in the HIV/AIDS struggle. The place gave us a creative space, allowed us to be in touch with God's creation, to experience and to see and hear God's creative hand anew in the New Year and within our environment. We did frightfully, pleasantly and awesomely come to fellowship with frogs, snakes, scorpions, zebras, giraffes, elephants, water hogs, the eland, the green trees, mountains and valleys—as we struggled with the question of how the church could effectively become the bearers of God's will for creation in the HIV/AIDS era. It became a special time for our own spiritual restoration, excellent fellowship and intellectual stimulation of a rare kind; as we read, debated and commented on each other's work. One thing became very clear: we became aware of how rare this discussion on HIV/AIDS is within our own communities of worship and work. Given the intensity of our discussions, we even saw potential in putting up a book on *Re-reading the Bible in the HIV/AIDS Context,* using the passages that we analyzed.

Generally, our quest was: How can the church break the silence and the stigma surrounding HIV/AIDS, and take every given opportunity to heal our hurting communities by being active partners in HIV/AIDS prevention, the provision of quality care, and in the mitigation of its impact? We believe that the resources of the church: its scriptures, its liturgy, its values, its members, its leaders and its buildings, are powerful weapons and resources for energizing and awakening the church to play its role effectively in the fight against HIV/AIDS. Our nine months of work has finally come to completion, compiled under the title, *AfricaPraying: A Handbook of HIV/AIDS Sensitive Sermons and Liturgy.*

To dwell a little on the title, 'Africa praying' describes a Christian church that knows God as the author of all life; as a God who cares for all; as a God who bestows upon each human being the dignity of bearing God's image; as a God who gives each of us the right to enjoy the resources of the earth; as a God who gives all of us the responsibility of leadership and decision making in keeping the earth and everything in it good. 'Africa praying' describes a justice seeking church that actively seeks to liberate God's created world from all forms of oppression, including HIV/AIDS. 'Africa praying' is a compassionate church that moves, like prophet Ezekiel descending into the valley of dry bones, to plant hope in a hopelessness people. We, the writers of these sermon guidelines, hope that many church leaders, workers, members, Sunday school teachers, Bible study and worship leaders, will immerse themselves in this resource and emerge strengthened and renewed to fight a good fight in healing our hurting families, friends, churches, communities, countries, continent, and indeed in healing the world as a whole. Towards this end, I commend you to the Spirit of power and fire as you become active partners with God in the struggle against HIV/AIDS, and against all forms of oppression that mar the beauty of creation.

Professor Musa W. Dube,
HIV/AIDS and Theological Consultant, Ecumenical HIV/AIDS Initiative.
July 28, 2003, Gaborone, Botswana.

Part 1
Services for Life Markers

1. Birthdays
        Matthew 2:1-15 (Musa W. Dube)
        Exodus 2:1-10 (Augustine C. Mosupole)
        Exodos 2:1-10 (Felicidade N. Cherinda)

2. Confirmations
        I Samuel 1:1-28 (Isabel Apawo Phiri)

3. Weddings
        Genesis 1:26-31 (Isabel Apawo Phiri)
        Genesis 1:26-31 and 3:15-24 (Isabel Apawo Phiri)

4. Anniversaries
        Exodus 12:1-14 (Isabel Apawo Phiri)

5. Graduations and Closing Ceremonies
        Jeremiah 5:17 (Musa W. Dube)

6. Death and Funerals
        Luke 7:11-17 (Isabel Apawo Phiri)
        John 11:1-44 (Moiseraele P. Dibeela)
        Luke 8:22-25 (Augustine C. Musopule)

7. Tomb Unveilings
        I Corinthians 15:35-58 (Ezra Chitando)

8. Healing and Memorial Services
        Psalm 23 (Musa W. Dube and Faluta L. Moyo)

9. Thanksgiving
        I Chronicles 29:10-19 (Tinyiko S. Maluleke)
        Revelations 2:1-7 (Moiseraele P. Dibeela)
        I Chronicles 29:10-19 (Felicidade N. Cherinda)

1. Birthdays

BIRTHDAYS AND CELEBRATIONS OF LIFE
Sermon Text: Matthew 2:1-15

In preparation, get drummers, arrange for ululation, assign different readers for the different parts, ask the choir/youth rappers or poets to present the song (Jabulani) in their own artistic mode and tune. In addition, the stage or meeting place may be arranged to underline the celebration of life using relevant objects (green trees, flowers, grains of corn, etc.) from your social context and denominational background. If you come from a tradition that does not use written liturgy, you may go straight to the sermon. The service may be used specifically for a birthday or for celebrating life in general.

Call to Worship

Drums of celebration for the opening

Leader 1:	Praise be to you, Son of God; When you were endangered; When you were a child; You found refuge in Africa. (Matthew 2:13-15)
Leader 2:	Praise be to you, Son of God; When you were crucified; When the cross was too heavy for you; You found help from an African, Simon of Cyrene. (Luke 23:26)
Leader 3:	Praise be to you, Son of God; When you taught the early church about your mission to all; When you sought to teach Phillip that your Gospel is for all; You sent the Ethiopian Eunuch to him. (Acts 8:26-40)
Leader 4:	Praise be to you, Son of God; You were always with us here in Africa; Where you grew in wisdom and the fear of God; You were with us in your suffering; You were with us when you reached out to the whole world.
Leader 5:	Praise be to you, Son of God; You are Emmanuel, the God with us; (Matthew 1:23) You will never leave us or forsake us; (Hebrews 13:5) Even today as we speak you dwell in Africa; Crucified with us in all our tribulations and rising with us in our joys.
The Celebrant/s:	You have been with me/us from the beginning; And you will be always with me/us.

3

Women and men ululate in praise of God, in joy, thanksgiving for God's love and for protection of our lives in Africa, and the lives of the celebrants.

Song
Jabulani Africa

Jabulani, Africa, Inkosi ikhona (2x) // Rejoice Africa, the Lord Liveth
Jabulani lonke, Jabulani Sizwe (2x) // May you all rejoice, Rejoice you nations
Jabulani, Jabulani (6x) // Rejoice, Rejoice
Jabulani lonke Jabulani Sizwe (2x) // May you all rejoice, Rejoice you nations

Jabula Mama lo Baba, Inkosi ikhona (2x) // Rejoice mother & father, the Lord Liveth
Jabula sisi (Malome), Jabula Bhudi (anti) Rejoice sister, Rejoice brother
Jabulani, Jabulani (6x) // Rejoice, Rejoice
Jabulani lonke, Jabulani Sizwe (2x) // May you all rejoice, Rejoice you nations

Jabulani Botswana, Jabula Zimbabwe // Rejoice Botswana, Rejoice Zimbabwe
Jabula Namibia, Jabula Lesotho // Rejoice Namibia, Rejoice Lesotho
Jabula Zambia, Jabula Azania // Rejoice Zambia, Rejoice Azania
Jabulani lonke, Jabulani sizwe (2x) // May you all rejoice, Rejoice you nations

Jabulani Angola, Jabula Mozambique // Rejoice Angola, Rejoice Mozambique
Jabula Malawi, Jabula Tanzania // Rejoice Malawi, Rejoice Tanzania
Jabula Congo, Jabula Kenya // Rejoice Congo, Rejoice Kenya
Jabulani Jabulani (6x) // Rejoice, Rejoice (6x)
Jabulani lonke, Jabulani sizwe (2x) // May you all rejoice, Rejoice you nations

Jabula Ghana, Jabula Somalia // Rejoice Ghana, Rejoice Somalia
Jabula Gabon, Jabula Senegal // Rejoice Gabon, Rejoice Senegal
Jabulani Tunisia, Jabula Swaziland // Rejoice Tunisia, Rejoice Swaziland
Jabulani, Jabulani (6x) // Rejoice, Rejoice
Jabulani lonke, Jabulani sizwe (2x) // May you all rejoice, Rejoice you nations

Jabulani Africa, Inkosi ikhona // Rejoice Africa, the Lord Liveth

(© Musa W. Dube)

Introduction

The HIV/AIDS epidemic's attack on life has brought us to be more thankful for each day that we live. It brings us to be more aware that life is a gift from God and that we should celebrate it; we should value and protect it. While in the past, the increasingly youth oriented world led some to hide their actual age, or to regret getting old, HIV/AIDS has brought a change. Now whenever one sees a very old woman or man walking with a stick, one stops with awesome wonder and appreciation, knowing how blessed this person has been to be given the opportunity to live for so long. With the HIV/AIDS epidemic, it is no longer guaranteed that one will live to this stage of aging. The fact that life expectancy has fallen from the 65-70 years down to 42-32, speaks for itself. Now each birthday is special and each new year is seen for what it is—a great and real blessing of life. One has been protected. One is being given another opportunity to live. A birthday is therefore, a special occasion to thank God for life, to celebrate life, to ask for more blessings, and to acknowledge those who care for one's wellbeing—parents, friends, God and national leaders.

In Matthew 2:1-15, it is Jesus' birthday. Some come to celebrate, such as the wise men from the east. But we are also brought face to face with an endangered life. Herod seeks to eliminate this child. God intervenes by sending a dream to the wise men and an angel to the parents. The parents act. They flee to Egypt where Jesus grows up safely, until the death of Herod. Each one of us has a birthday, hence a time to reflect on God's protection, parental care, the encouragement of friends, hospitable countries, and to be thankful for the gift of life, as well as to acknowledge that we have a duty to stay alive.

We Listen to the Word of God

Reading of the text: Matthew 2:1-15.

DETAILS OF THE TEXT
Verse 1-2:
➤ These verses give both the time (the time of King Herod) and place (Bethlehem of Judea) as the setting of the Jesus' birth story. But it also introduces key characters: Jesus, King Herod, the wise men from the East, and the Jews.

➤ Note two factors: Both Herod and Jesus are introduced as kings, hence planting the seed for potential conflict.

➤ Note that while Jesus is identified as "King of Jews," non-Jews, the wise men from the east (Asia), "come to pay him homage," indicating that he will be king of all people.

➤ Note: "We have seen his star at its rising," indicating he will be a light to the world. But more importantly, each person, and each child's birth is tantamount to a new star rising into the world and into our lives. We must see and acknowledge this star, celebrate it and allow it to light our world and lives—for each person is made in God's image and in each person there is God's breath (Genesis 1:27 and 2:7).

Verse 3-6:
➤ King Herod is naturally threatened to hear that another king has come into his own domain! He gathers his own intelligence to verify the information. They confirm his worst fears: in Bethlehem there, "shall come a ruler who is to shepherd my people Israel."

➤ Underline that we are born in a world of many evils: political powers, economic deprivations, wars, diseases, drugs, and many other factors that threaten the gift of life given to us. Jesus himself was not exempted.

Verse 7-8:
➤ Herod takes a second step. He confers with the wise men, collecting more information—he wants, "the exact time when the star had appeared." Then he says to them, "Go and search

diligently for the child; and when you have found him, bring me word so that I may also go and pay him homage."

➤ Highlight that the forces of evil that attack lives are quite deliberate and quite informed about us. They sometimes search for us. Our intent to protect life must be equally intentional.

Verse 9-10:
➤ The well wishers of Jesus journey to find him.

➤ Note that the star guides them, leading them to where the child was.

➤ Highlight that unlike Herod and his intelligence, they are "overwhelmed with joy."

➤ Underline that people who wish us well, can see the star that God put in us, they can see God's image in us, and they are happy for us.

Verses 11-12:
➤ These verses are very important. The child is in the full presence of all who care: the mother, the wise men and God, who directs the latter away from Herod.

➤ Highlight that the wise men from the east (Asia) are the first to pay homage (worship Jesus). They knelt down and worshiped him. This is an early indication that the mission of Jesus is the story of God reaching out to both Jews, and all people of the world.

➤ Highlight how the well-wishers opened their "treasure chests" and "offered him gifts of gold, frankincense and myrrh," all of which were expensive gifts. Underline how those who care for us, give to us from "their treasure chests" the very best that they have. These gifts need not be just materialistic as the next verse indicates. It could be in the form of words, wisdom, guidance, counseling, encouragement, and affirmation of the stars that they see shining in us and above us.

➤ Consequently the well-wishers do not return to Herod, who is not a well-wisher. They return to their country through another road, for Herod seeks the child not to worship him or give him the best gifts, but to kill the child. Consequently, Herod never saw the star of this child.

➤ Underline the role of friends and well wishers to protect the celebrants from danger—to take another road; to refuse to become informants of evil powers.

Verse 13-15:
➤ These verses are notable for the role of God and parents in protecting our lives. God speaks to parents informing them about the dangers surrounding the child and calling them to protect the child. God speaks and the parents act.

➤ They flee to Egypt and remain there until Herod is no longer alive—until the child is no longer in danger, and then they return (2:19-23). This underlines the need and the important role of parents to cooperate with God in protecting the lives of their children. A birthday is therefore also a time to celebrate parents.

- Highlight the role of Egypt as a hospitable country to an endangered life. Given the amount of political and economic refugees/displaced people we have in Africa, the role of Egypt in welcoming and protecting Christ remains quite critical in today's world.

- But the fact that Jesus was born a king of Jews, greeted and worshipped by wise men from the east (Asia), and fled and found refuge in Egypt (Africa), underlines that he was a Messiah/Christ of all. But it also underlines that we are interconnected and our health as a world will depend on many actors from different continents and countries.

- Underline, that in this HIV/AIDS era every child and every person's life is endangered. We are however, looking for well wishers, caring parents, hospitable countries and God's voice, to celebrate and protect the lives of those we love and of our children. We are challenged to see God's star leading us to the presence of each child and to hear God leading us away from all that endangers them.

We Apply the Word of God to Ourselves

WHAT CAN WE LEARN?
- That at all times life is threatened, even Christ's life was threatened;
- That we also have support from God, parents, friends and other countries;
- That birthdays are a good time to celebrate life and God's protection;
- That we need to see the star—God's image and breath in each person.

WHAT DO WE HAVE TO CONFESS?
- That we have sometimes been the source of danger to life;
- That we sometimes fail to see God's star upon all people;
- That we often fail to give our very best gifts to the children who are born to us;
- That we are sometimes unworthy friends, parents and countries;
- That as friends, sometimes we do not give the best gifts to others.

WHAT CAN WE BE THANKFUL FOR?
- For God's gift of life and protection;
- For supporting friends, caring parents and hospitable countries;
- For God's salvation that was extended to all people and continents.

WHAT CAN WE PRAY FOR?
- For God's protection against political leaders who endanger life;
- For countries that will receive those who are political refugees (displaced people);
- For parents and friends to protect the lives of those they love;
- For every birthday celebrant to realize they have the responsibility to stay alive, especially as they confront HIV/AIDS.

We Apply the Word of God to the Congregation

WHAT CAN WE FEEL?
- Grateful that we are not alone whenever our lives are endangered.

WHAT CAN WE BE?
- A hospitable, supportive and parenting church and country.

WHAT CAN WE DO?
- Set up services for displaced people/refugees;
- Work with NGOs who support displaced people;
- Speak out and act on behalf of those whose life is endangered;
- Take the fight against HIV/AIDS as our responsibility in protecting life.

Conclusion: A Word on Society

Society is full of many different players, in so far as protecting life is concerned. How is your society? What about your political leaders? Do they protect and celebrate the lives of all? Sometimes this is not the case—the stars of life cease to shine in the presence of murderous political leaders. What is the attitude of your country towards displaced people? The church is called to walk with all God's people in protecting each person and celebrating their lives as God given. It must call out and act to see to it that life is protected, especially in the HIV/AIDS era. It must also challenge governments to be hospitable to displaced people.

Song
Rea mo leboga // We give our thanks (Thuma Mina, No. 108)

Closing Prayer for the Celebrant/s
The word of the Lord says to you:
"Before I formed you in the womb I knew you,
And before you were born, I consecrated you,
I appointed you a prophet to the nations." (Jeremiah 1:5)

Ululation
In praise and thanks of God for life and protection

Suggested objects/symbols/ideas: A key holder, wrapped present/s to give, pebbles/words to exchange with all participants as a pledge of friendship and care.

By Musa W. Dube

BIRTHDAYS
Sermon Text: Exodus 2:1-10

Introduction

Preparing for the birth of a baby is a discrete affair, and in Malawi cultures, is accompanied by fear of the potential dangers. These days HIV/AIDS is an immediate danger, especially because it can be transmitted from mother to child. In Malawi, a pregnancy is referred to as a sickness and delivery as a healing. As if this is not enough, the little bundle of human life must be protected medically and magically to ward off any hostile force against it, or the family. Call it immunization if you will. The medicines or protective charms are worn around the neck, the waist, wrists and ankles. We are all responsible to preserve and protect life. It is an evil world into which we are born. Life is full of dangers, and whether we survive or not is up to God. All this gives cause for celebration when life continues, and when the individual keeps adding years as they grow up towards responsible adulthood.

Birthday celebrations or observations of life markers are significant for the individual, the family and the entire clan, because suffering and death diminishes clan strength and possibilities for survival. All that we can do in vulnerable times is to take precautions and wait in faith. This is what the parents of Moses did. Some of the practical steps that can be taken are: prevention of transmission of the virus from mother to child, caring for those who are already sick, and protecting children from the various dangers to their lives, including contracting HIV/AIDS through sexual abuse, early sexual activity and through providing life skills education.

We Listen to the Word of God

We note in this passage the danger that Moses faced as a child. What dangers do children face today, especially in view of the HIV/AIDS pandemic?

Moses' mother, sister and midwives intervened strategically in the protection of Hebrew children, including Moses. What steps can you as individuals and faith communities take to protect children from the dangers you have mentioned?

What moved Pharaoh's daughter to act in the way she did? What role is there for other people to intervene in the lives of our children globally?

DETAILS OF THE TEXT
Verses 2-4:
➢ Out of desperation the parents hide the child, they will do anything to protect it and save it.

Verse 5-6:
➢ Pharaoh's daughter was aware of her father's decree and she guessed that the baby was a Hebrew, and yet she was moved by something beyond class, politics, ethnicity and gender to feel compassion.

Verses 7-10:
➤ The sister provided timely and appropriate intervention and saw that her brother was adopted and cared for by her own mother. She influenced life changing decisions with small steps and timely suggestions.

We Apply God's Word to Ourselves and to the Congregation

WHAT CAN WE LEARN?
- That God is the only giver and protector of our lives.
- Any birthday celebration among Christians should be regarded as a time of deep reflection on the way in which God not only brings a new life into this world, but also protects it and makes it grow, in spite of the hostile environment in which we live.
- A birthday celebration should be regarded as a privileged time for us to think about the miraculous ways in which God brings us this world.
- A birthday is a good moment for us to reflect on how to care for life and protect it, especially the lives of our children.
- We can pray, "So teach us to number our days that we may acquire a heart of wisdom" (Psalms 90:12).

WHAT CAN WE CONFESS?
- Failure to celebrate our lives when we are faced with life threatening situations;
- Celebrating in the wrong way by not focusing often on the giver of life; (Job 1:5)
- That as men we endanger children, through war and sexual violence;
- Failure to take the necessary steps to protect life endangered by HIV/AIDS.

WHAT CAN WE BE THANKFUL FOR?
- That whether we are already old, or are still young, and whatever our health, social and economic situation, when we are given another year, or even another day to live in this world, we should be thankful to God and celebrate God's gift and protection of life in us. Let us remind ourselves that God's grace is always sufficient and that God's power is made complete in weakness. (Read II Corinthians 12:9)
- That we also have the opportunity to save the lives of those who are endangered.
- For women who care for children.

WHAT CAN WE PRAY FOR?
- That God gives us ability to celebrate our lives even in threatening situations. Let's remind ourselves of what the Psalmist says, "You prepare a table for me in the presence of my enemies". (Psalms 23:5)
- For orphans who celebrate their birthdays without their parents and for those supporting the orphans.
- The ability to act like Pharoah's daughter and Moses' sister, who ensured that the child grew up under good care.

WHAT CAN WE FEEL?
- Angry at those who use their power to oppress, discriminate and destroy life;
- Concern for children in areas of conflict who have been maimed;
- Love and compassion for the midwives, Moses' mother, sister and Pharaoh's daughter.

WHAT SHOULD WE BE?
- People of love and compassion;
- Parents who protect children.

WHAT CAN WE DO?
- Resist oppression and uphold children's rights;
- Show concerned for all children's welfare;
- Protect children against rape and HIV/AIDS infection.

We Apply the Word of God to the Congregation and Society

Institutions and public figures have a lot of clout with which to influence public policy for good. They can make a difference in the lives of one or many, even in matters of life and death. Moses was sentenced to death even before he was born. Had Pharaoh's daughter and other players not acted, Moses would have been as good as dead.

- Discuss with the congregation or church committee about situations in which you or your congregation can make a difference for children, especially ways to mitigate the effects of HIV/AIDS and in order to save lives condemned by evil forces to death?

- How can your congregation influence public policy in relation to family, local community, national and global needs in the light of the HIV/AIDS?

- What is the relationship between dangers threatening children and global causes of poverty?

- All the players in this story made a difference. Draw up a plan of action on ways to make a difference to children in your community, so that birthday celebrations can be what they are meant to be: a community looking to the future with hope for Africa's children.

Song
Sing any traditional happy birthday song for those who are celebrating their birthdays this week or month.

Prayer
God of love, God of compassion,
In the midst of death and evil,
You mercifully look after us:
Protecting, providing, and smiling,
Constantly reassuring us of your care.
Grant to us the joy of this occasion,
Especially as we celebrate our birthdays
Knowing that your love is life.

Teach us to number our days aright
That we may acquire a heart of wisdom
Through Him whose life
Has become our light, even Jesus Christ.
Amen

Suggested objects/symbols/ideas: Cradle, basket, photo album, seed or seedling.

By Augustine C. Musopule

NASCIMENTO
Texto Sugerido: Êxodos 2:1-10

Oração

Obrigado Senhor por nos ter reunido para em conjunto contemplarmos a tua glória. Obrigado pelo dom desta nova vida. Ela vem ressuscitar as nossas esperanças, de que a vida ainda é possível, apesar de muita morte que contemplamos cada dia. Senhor, ajude-nos a criar esta criança no teu conhecimento, na justiça e no amor ao próximo. Dê-lhe a sabedoria de se afastar de tudo quanto lhe possa ser prejudicial, e que saiba se proteger contra o HIV/SIDA. Pedimos isso tudo em nome do nosso Senhor Jesus Cristo.

Introdução

Com muita tristeza constatamos que nos dias de hoje, o nascimento de uma criança deixou de ser motivo de alegria em muitas famílias. As causas da falta de alegria são várias. Dentre elas podemos citar as seguintes: Fome, doença, imaturidade dos progenitores, guerras, violação e outras. Constatamos que apesar da existência de Direitos Internacionais de proteção à criança, em muitos casos ,ou não são conhecidos ou não são respeitados. Em África, diariamente tomamos conhecimento de assissinato de bebés recém nascidos pelas próprias mães que lhes atiram nas latas de lixo, nas drenagens e outros lugares inimagináveis. Outras crianças são abandonadas nas maternidades, algumas nascem infectadas pelo vírus do HIV/SIDA, outras morrem de sarampo,outras ficam órfãs de pai e mãe, outras são violadas por pessoas adultas imorais com o pretexto de curar SIDA e muitas outras morrem de fome e vivem estigmatizadas. As ameaças à vida não são um fenómeno novo. O texto mostra claramente o que aconteceu com Moisés. O próprio Jesus não escapou à condenação logo após o seu nascimento (Mt. 2: 13). Porém, em todas essas histórias, as crianças foram salvas porque Deus agiu. Nos nossos dias, Deus continua a agir. O que precisamos é de união e solidariedade entre as famílias, e entre os dirigentes dos nossos países na proteção das nossas crianças contra todas as formas da morte e de perigos.

Escutemos a Palavra de Deus

Leia o texto, sublinhe com um lápis as palavras mais importantes. Tente compreender a sua estrutura.

DETALHES
V.1 Levi:
➤ Um dos doze filhos de Jacó e uma das doze tribos de Israel. O texto sugere que o casamento efectuou-se entre as tribos de Israel.

VV.2-4:
➤ Nascimento de uma criança e a luta travada para conservá-la com vida.

VV.5-6:
➤ A intervenção divina através da filha de Faraó.

VV.7-10:
➤ A criança é salva e criada por duas mães: Uma biológica e outra adoptiva.

A Palavra de Deus para nós.

QUE PODEMOS APRENDER?
• Que Deus nunca abandona as suas criaturas quer elas estejam ou não conscientes disso;
• Que muitas vezes Deus utiliza as forças a Ele hostis para a realização dos seus desígnios;
• Que tipo de perigos as crianças enfrentam nos nossos dias?

QUE TEMOS DE CONFESSAR?
• Que muitas vezes esquecemos de convidar Deus quando fazemos planos da nossa vida;
• Que muitas vezes somos culpados pela morte de crianças.

EM QUE DEVEMOS ESTAR GRATOS A DEUS?
• Pelo facto de Deus nos ensinar permanentemente a escolher, a lutar e a amar a vida.

QUE PODEMOS PEDIR NAS NOSSAS ORAÇÕES?
• Pelo amor, respeito, paz, justiça e solidariedade entre as pessoas;
• Pela valorização da vida e pelo conhecimento de Deus.

A Palavra de Deus para a Sociedade

A vida é uma dádiva de Deus. Contudo, tem se verificado que muita gente não dá o devido valor a ela. Isso é demonstrado pelos hábitos nocivos que consciente ou incoscientemente as pessoas adquirem e praticam. Dentre esses hábitos podemos citar o uso e consumo abusivos de álccol, de drogas, a violação de menores,etc. Além dessas práticas, o mundo e em especial a Àfrica Sub Sahariana, debate-se hoje com a pandemia do HIV/SIDA. Esta doença não é um castigo de Deus contra pecadores como muitos propagam. Deus é amor e não se contenta com a morte de ninguém (Ez. 18.31c). No passado existiram muitas doenças que mataram muitas pessoas. Ex: a varíola, a febre tifóide, a lepra, a tubrculose, etc. Hoje em dia, essas doenças já não matam porque existem medicamentos para a sua cura. Não há, por isso, lugar para discriminar aqueles que vivem com o vírus. O que é necessário é que todos vivam em harmonia e que se continue a trabalhar até se encontrar medicamentos. Para travar o seu alastramento, é preciso seguir as instruções que nos são transmitidas através de organismos competentes. Cientistas, doentes e toda a sociedade devem estar unidos contra esta doença. É preciso que a força e vontade de viver esteja no coração de cada um de nós. Devemos ter fé de que Deus está connosco como esteve com a mãe e a irmã de Moisés no Egipto. Deus está sempre do lado daqueles que lutam contra os Faraós de todos os tempos.

Canção
Escolher uma canção que esteja de acordo com o tema

Oração
Deus de amor e de compaixão, aproximamo-nos a ti, cheios de pesar e de vergonha, porque não somos capazes, de compreender que nos amas acima de tudo. O nosso sentimento é de que vivemos debaixo da sombra da morte. È nos difícil compreender que já nos tiraste de lá, e que esperas de nós uma atitude que demonstra fé e confiança na vida eterna prometida por Jesus. Não nos abandone, antes nos guie nos caminhos de esperança de que um dia, África conhecerá e viverá na paz, na saúde e na prosperidade, pela graça e pela misericórdia que nos são dadas pelo Teu Filho Jesus Cristo e pelo Espírito Santo. Amen

Suggested objects: Fotografia de um casal olhando com amor para o seu bebé, um berço com um bebé deitado, uma criança dando um beijo a um bebé, etc.

Por: Felicidade N. Cherinda

2. Confirmation

SERVICE ON CONFIRMATION/DEDICATION
Sermon Texts: I Samuel 1:1-28

Prayer
Thank you God that every good and perfect gift comes from you. Thank you for the blessing that children are. As we dedicate this child to you, we pray that you will bless her/him so that she/he will grow in stature, in wisdom and in favour with God and people. Help the parents to bring her/him up in the fear and knowledge of the Lord. We pray in Jesus' name, Amen

Song (Chichewa)
Ndidzakutamandani Mulungu wanga, Halleluyah!
(I will praise you my God)
Ndizakutamandani Mulungu wanga
(I will praise you my God)
Mwachita zazikulu pamoyo wanga, Halleluyah!
(You have done great things in my life)
Ndizakutamandani Mulungu wanga
(I will praise you my God)
(repeat)
(A Malawian Community Song)

Introduction

Confirmation/dedication is a very important time in the lives Christian parents and their children. It is a time when the parents make a public declaration to bring up their child in the fear and knowledge of the Lord. It is also a time when a person who was baptized as an infant makes a public declaration that she/he is making a personal commitment to God, in the presence of a worshiping community. Today, this commitment is made in the context of many challenges, which include the existence of the HIV/AIDS pandemic. Children are a blessing from God and need to be cared for. As part and parcel of caring for our children, we need to do everything within our power to protect our children from contracting HIV/AIDS. If the parents are already infected, they need to think seriously before they decide to conceive a child. At birth, medication should be taken to reduce mother to child transmission of the virus. As the children grow, parents also have the responsibility of giving them accurate knowledge about the virus and how they can protect themselves from getting infected with HIV.

We Listen to the Word of God

Read the sermon texts:1 Samuel 1:1-28. This can be done by the leader or a member of the congregation. Mark the important words with a pencil.

Samuel was dedicated to God after his mother weaned him. He served God for the rest of his life and he brought tremendous reforms in Israel, even in the days when Israel had no king and everyone was doing what they saw fit.

DETAILS OF THE TEXT

Verses 1-8:
➤ Samuel was born in a polygamous Hebrew family. His father was Elkanah and his mother was Hannah. Samuel's parents were worshipping people. Shiloh was the main worshiping place for Israel at the time. Hannah was a very unhappy person because she could not conceive. In the Hebrew times, just like in traditional Africa, barrenness was a humiliation.

Verses 9-18:
➤ Hannah prayed for a child and promised to dedicate him to God. God answered Hannah's prayer, also as a special provision for the salvation of the Hebrews. He was to be a Nazirite. The rules governing a Nazirite are found in Numbers 6. The major difference is that in the case of Samuel, his status as a Nazirite was permanent.

Verse 19-28:
➤ Samuel was dedicated to God by his mother and by the priest Eli. Despite the fact that Samuel's mother had no any other children at the time of Samuel's dedication, she fulfilled her promise to God by taking Samuel to live at the Temple in Shiloh.

-

We Apply the Word of God to Ourselves

WHAT CAN WE LEARN?
- God is able to provide a child to a barren person;
- God listens to the prayers of the oppressed;
- When a person makes a vow to God, it should be fulfilled even if it means giving up what one wanted badly;
- Polygamy contributes to disharmony in a marriage relationship;
- God values women even when they are barren.

WHAT DO WE HAVE TO CONFESS?
- Do we value children more than the women who are not able to give birth?
- Do we confess that in today's world polygamy can promote the spread of HIV/AIDS?
- Do we fulfill the promises we have made to God?
- Have we fulfilled our responsibility in teaching our children about HIV/AIDS?
- Do you confess that our insistence on child bearing hinders HIV/AIDS prevention?
- Do you confess that we have not helped orphaned children?

WHAT CAN WE BE THANKFUL FOR?
- Life, whether we have children or not;
- The children that God has entrusted to us to bring up in the fear and knowledge of the Lord;
- That God has entrusted us as parents with the responsibility to teach our children about HIV/AIDS;
- That we need to realize there are many orphaned children who need our parenting.

WHAT CAN WE PRAY FOR?
- Parents to take up their responsibility to bring up children in the knowledge and fear of the Lord;
- Parents to love their children enough to teach them about HIV/AIDS and how to prevent infections;
- Parents to love their children even when they are infected with HIV;
- Church members to become parents to orphaned children.

We Apply the Word of God to the Congregation

WHAT CAN WE FEEL?
- Happy that children are a gift from God;
- Sad that some children have died of AIDS because we did not take up our
- responsibility to teach them about HIV;
- Guilty for not keeping our promises to God;
- Sorry for not loving women who are barren;
- Repentant that we are not bothered about the welfare of orphaned children.

WHAT CAN WE BE?
- Members of the congregation who accept the responsibility to teach all the children of our congregation about HIV/AIDS;

- Members of the congregation who will fulfill the promises that they made to God;
- A congregation that does not discriminate against women who are barren;
- A congregation that makes a programmatic response to orphaned children.

WHAT CAN WE DO?
- Teach about HIV/AIDS in our congregation, children's church, youth meetings etc.;
- Be inclusive of mothers and barren women in all our church activities;
- Start church programs for fostering, adopting and helping orphans.

Conclusion: A Word on Society

Parents sometimes struggle to have children, and whatever choices they make affect the children either positively or negatively. In the era of HIV/AIDS, to choose polygamy as a solution to bareness is to choose death.

Hannah expressed her devotion to the Lord by dedicating her son Samuel to full a promise that she had made to the Lord. Christian parents today may express their commitment to God by giving their sons and daughters to the HIV/AIDS ministry or the work of missions. Those parents who continue to encourage, support and pray for their children will find great favor with God. We can also extend our parenthood to include children who have lost a parent due to HIV/AIDS.

Prayer of Commitment

To be said by the whole congregation.

Lord we commit ourselves to be your hands in our societies. We commit ourselves to bear the good news of knowledge about HIV/AIDS to members of our families and the communities where we live. We commit ourselves not to discriminate against barren women but to show them love and compassion. We commit ourselves to be caring to orphaned children. We pray that you give us the courage to do what we know is right. In Jesus' name, Amen

Song

What the Lord has done for me,
I cannot tell it all, (3X)
He saved me and washed me in his blood.

So I will sing Halleluyah,
I will shout Halleluyah,
I will sing, shout, Praise the Lord. (2x)
(Popular Song)

Benediction
May the Lord keep and guide you.

Symbols/objects and commitments: Beads, gifts, water, candles, testimonies from barren women and a youth about the goodness of remaining in the teachings of God, testimonies from child-headed homes, orphans and elders caring for orphans, and musical instruments.

By Isabel Apawo Phiri

3. Weddings

WEDDINGS: PARTNERSHIP IN MARRIAGE
Sermon Text: Genesis 1:26-31

Introduction

Weddings are still common occurrences in spite of the HIV/AIDS epidemic in Sub-Saharan Africa. I have chosen the theme of partnership in this passage, as I believe it is a very important component of a fulfilling and lasting marriage. This theme is especially important for Botswana, and most other African countries, where it is often difficult to talk about partnership within marriage relationships because culture, law, the society and the church discriminate against women. The Bible has often been abused and misinterpreted to perpetuate this subordination of women. Research has proven that the impact of the unequal position of women in relation to their male counterparts has had a direct influence on the spread of HIV/AIDS. The gender disparities have manifested themselves, in that women are sexually powerless. They are more open and vulnerable to sexual abuse, exploitation and harassment. Research findings suggest that we have to address the issue of gender inequality in relationships in order to address the consequences and the impact of HIV/AIDS. It is this theme of partnership that we as ministers ought to encourage in our contact with couples, since it is often the inequality of genders that weakens the partnership relationship in marriage. Faithfulness, respect and communication are all pillars through which the partnership relationship could be affirmed.

We Listen to the Word of God

DETAILS OF THE TEXT

This beautiful passage reflects the strong partnership in relationship that ought to exist between two people in marriage. This creation story does not specify any positions of power between the two and there is no domination of one partner over the other. Instead it emphasizes common support and equal responsibility. Both partners reflect the image of their Creator. The author of Genesis does not set any specialized roles and responsibilities for each partner, only that there are two varieties namely, man and the woman. This is often an ideal model of partnership set for marriage. It is not easy to achieve such partnership today, yet an important one to strive for if one wants to have a long and successful marriage. This is because as I have indicated above, our traditions and laws have set ranks of power. Our society and Church has set gender roles and responsibilities, and we often believe that those are determinants of right and wrong within our marriage lives. These are strong influences in marriage life, particularly at home. We are influenced to believe that what is expected from ones culture or family it is how it should be. This is not to say that one should totally disregard those around you, but that the ultimate value of the partnership rests with the mutual support and equal partnership shared by the two. It is only when two people appreciate each other that they can appreciate the creation of God and their purpose for the world.

We Apply the Word of God to Ourselves

WHAT CAN WE LEARN?
- That we are each uniquely created in the image of God;
- That we are each important as human beings and have a specific purpose to fulfill;
- That we are responsible and have the ability to shape the partnership within marriage;
- That both men and women were blessed by God and given equal access to earthly resources.

WHAT DO WE HAVE TO CONFESS?
- That we often want to follow our own mind, instead of considering our partners in the relationship and therefore disregarding the partnership;
- That we are guilty of perpetuating the same discriminating language and attitude as
- the rest of the society against women;
- That God, the Creator of partnership, is often excluded in our marriages;
- That not honouring partnership has resulted in many incidences of abuse, unfaithfulness and the infection of women and men.
- That we have denied women access to property and leadership hence exposing them to high HIV/AIDS infection.

WHAT CAN WE BE THANKFUL FOR?
- For the many lifelong partnership relationships, and for people who strive for equal partnership in marriage;
- For men who do not treat women as inferior, but as their partners;
- For laws and NGO's that seek to empower women in society.

WHAT CAN WE PRAY FOR?
- That God gives us the wisdom and guidance to be sensitive to the needs of the other partner.
- That we would continue our partnership relationship in spite of poverty, unemployment and ill health, especially in the face of HIV/AIDS.
- That love in marriage might overcome all abuse, hurt and inequality.

We Apply the Word of God to our Church/Society

WHAT CAN WE DO?
- We can become agents of change to those laws and traditions that show favoritism to men.
- We can provide education so that men and women understand what partnership involves.
- We can provide a helping hand to couples that are in desperate need for advice, or need to restore their marriages.
- Actively engage in programs such as marriage counseling, pre-marital courses and family conflict resolution.

A Suggested Wedding Ceremony
Based on the theme of partnership in Genesis 1:26-31

Instead of the traditional practice where the father brings the bride and hands over his daughter (which seems to signify him handing over his 'responsibility/authority' to the groom), both parties enter the Church from different sides followed by the families.

Minister:	We are here today because (insert name of bride) and (insert name of groom) have decided of their own free will, that they would like to become partners in marriage.

Suggested objects/symbols: African baskets could be used to put bread and fruits. A basin and water with a hand towel can be used during the service.

Vows

Minister:	Do you (bride), take (groom) to be your spouse in marriage? Do you (groom) take (bride) to be your spouse in marriage?
Bride:	*Breaks the bread and feeds the groom* All I have I will share with you.
Groom:	*Breaks the bread and feeds the bride* All I have I will share with you.
Bride:	*Washes the grooms hands and dries them with the hand towel* I will always take care of you.
Groom:	*Washes the brides hands and dries them with the hand towel* I will also take care of you.

Exchange of rings

Bride:	My love will be your love.
Groom:	And my love will be your love.

The following words can be said whilst beads are exchanged
I will always respect your body. I will do my best to protect you from the infection of HIV/AIDS, but if it happens despite our effort, then you will still be mine and I will be yours till death parts us.

As a sign of the partnership between the families, The bride hands over a basket of fruit to the groom's parents, and the groom hands over a basket of fruits to the bride's parents. The parents do the same to the bride and groom. The following or similar words could be said.

We exchange these baskets of fruits as a sign that we will take care of each other and of God's creation.

Prayer

Minister:	Let us come before our Loving Parent in whose image we are all created. God our Creator we give you thanks and praise.
Groom:	Please forgive us when we mar your image because of our shortcomings and lack of love. Restore and bless the image of you in our lives for Christ's sake.
Minister:	Thank you for creating and sustaining our world. We thank you for living creatures and for our daily bread and water.
Bride:	Please forgive us when we destroy and pollute your creation for our own selfish ends. Restore and bless the world that you have given us so that our partnership might extend to all of your creation.
Minister:	Thank you for seedtime and harvest and all the good in your creation.
Bride and Groom:	Bind us together O God so that we might become an inspiration to each other. Help us to understand each other, our strengths and our weaknesses and in doing so become strong partners in the extension of your kingdom here on earth. We especially pray that in the face of all difficulties such as ill health, unemployment and especially HIV/AIDS, in which many relationships crumble, that our partnership would never wane. Make us partners, we pray in Jesus name.
All:	God, Giver of Life, forgive us when we do not care for each other and when we do not share food and water with those who are hungry and thirsty. Make us your instruments to restore our world in justice and love so that you may again look on our world and see that it is good. We pray in the name of Jesus Christ. Amen

A Blessing for the Bride and Groom

Just as the Father, the Son and the Holy Spirit live in unity, may they live together in peace and love to the very end of their lives.

Song
Bind us Together Lord

Appropriate hymns could be incorporated, that would further emphasis the theme of partnership.

Suggested objects: Rings, beads, pictures/sculptures of animals hugging.

By Cheryl Dibeela

WEDDING/MARRIAGE
Sermon Texts: Genesis 1:26-31 and 3:15-24

Prayer

Leader: We have come together before God to celebrate the joining together of these two people.

All: We come before you Lord, to bear witness to the love.

Leader: Lord you blessed the first wedding in the Garden of Eden.

All: We stand in your presence with this couple in our Garden of Eden.

Song (Xhosa)

Masithi: Amen siyakudumisa // (Sing amen: Amen, we praise your name O Lord)
Masithi: Amen, siyakudumisa // (Sing amen: Amen, we praise your name O Lord)
Maisithi: Amen Bawo // (Sing amen: Amen Amen)
Amen Bawo // (Amen Amen)
Amen siyakudumisa // (Amen we praise your name O Lord)

(Thuma Mina, 168)

Introduction

A wedding ceremony is an occasion that allows two people who have agreed to live together as a couple, to officially declare to the community that the union they are now entering is legal and binding. There are different types of weddings depending on several factors, two of which are the culture and religion of the two people who are getting married.

Weddings can take place between two people, even when one or both of them are sick. In today's world one challenge for marriage is if an infected partner does not disclose the fact that they have HIV/AIDS. This is a tragedy which needs a solution. It may happen that one partner was either married before or had a relationship, and was infected. It is therefore important to encourage the two partners to be tested for HIV/AIDS and disclose the results to each other. It must be up to the uninfected partner to decide whether to go ahead with the wedding ceremony or not. If they decide to go on regardless of the status, they should be given counselling on the consequences, and on methods to avoid infecting their partner.

We Listen to the Word of God

A member of the congregation or the leader can read the texts.

Genesis 1:26-31 is the first Bible story on the creation of humanity. The people were given stewardship of all that was created. Genesis 3:15-24 is about the punishment given to humanity after the fall.

DETAILS OF THE TEXT
➢ It is important to note that the word 'man' in this passage denotes both male and female. This is shown in verse 26.

➢ "Let us make man" – the correct word for man in this verse is humankind. It is male and female together that makes up humanity.
➢ "Image" and "likeness" here are interchangeable. Both women and men reflect the image of God.
➢ "Image of God" refers to moral, intellectual and spiritual capacities.
➢ "Have dominion" indicates that both men and women are to be stewards of God's creation.

Genesis 3:15-24:
➢ "I will put enmity between you and the woman" refers to the continual enmity between Satan and humanity.
➢ "He will crush your head and you will strike his heel" symbolizes the continuing struggle between God and evil as it manifest itself in the hearts of people.
➢ However, throughout generations, there is a redemptive element to the punishment, which will come through the woman's seed.
➢ "Pains in childbearing" is a punishment that is unique to women. In Africa many women die during child birth due to lack of good medical facilities.
➢ Adam, in verse 17, refers to man and not to humanity, as in chapter 1 verse 26. Eve is the name given to the woman.
➢ "Painful toil" was supposed to be a punishment unique to men but in Africa, the toiling of the ground is a job mainly shared between men and women.
➢ "Returning to the ground" refers to death, which is also a shared punishment for all humanity and not for men only.
➢ "Mother of all the living" is a sign of hope for the continuity of the human race in the midst of punishments.
➢ "God made garments of skin" reflects God's power to provide, despite the punishment.
➢ "Banished from the garden" refers to humanity working very hard to fend for themselves. It is also banishment from the presence of God. Redemption is only through the seed of the woman.

We Apply the Word of God to the Couple

WHAT CAN WE LEARN?
● God created men and women equal;
● Women and men have equal moral and spiritual capacities and responsibilities;
● That life lived in God's presence is a life of peace and tranquility;
● Both man and woman sinned and were punished by God;
● Diseases and death came to humanity after the fall;
● Salvation from sin and suffering is for both woman and man, through Christ.

WHAT DO WE HAVE TO CONFESS?
● Have we been transparent to one another as couples?
● Have we discussed HIV before marriage?
● Are we in denial that leads us to lack of openness?
● Has there been companionship and partnership in our marriages?
● Is marriage considered a covenant?
● Many husbands have infected their wives through unfaithfulness.

WHAT CAN WE BE THANKFUL FOR?
- For God creating male and female to be partners and to complement each other;
- That with a clear understanding of God's will in marriage, a woman and man can protect each other from HIV/AIDS infection.

WHAT CAN WE PRAY FOR?
- That couples love each other enough to protect each other from HIV/AIDS. The fact that a couple is married does not rule out infection from HIV/AIDS.
- In particular, male partners are encouraged to be faithful even though African culture turns a blind eye to infidelity from married men.

The leader can bring testimonies of other couples.

We Apply the Word of God to the Congregation

WHAT CAN WE FEEL?
- Ashamed for not being honest with our marriage partners;
- Sorry for not discussing HIV/AIDS before marriage;
- Remorse for not condemning male unfaithfulness;
- Responsible for sentencing many faithful wives to death.

WHAT CAN WE BE?
- Congregations that promote honesty among couples;
- A caring community for those who are infected with HIV/AIDS;
- A supportive community to the couples that disclose their HIV/AIDS status;
- A church that advocates for women's empowerment in the HIV/AIDS context.

WHAT CAN WE DO?
- Do members of the congregation pledge to help the young couple to fulfill their vows?
- Hold seminars for married couples where they can openly discuss.

Conclusion: A Word on Society

In Africa, new HIV/AIDS infections are increasing mainly among married couples. This information points to the importance of couples maintaining their marriage vows. Misinterpretation of the creation story, leading woman to be seen as inferior to man, has not helped in curbing the HIV/AIDS epidemic. Deliberate infection of your partner and your children is committing murder. It is also important for husband and wife to take care of each other if they are already infected.

The verse instructing us to be fruitful and multiply is difficult in the context of HIV/AIDS. When a couple is HIV positive, precautions need to be taken before having children. Where treatment is available to stop mother to child transmission of HIV, this should be taken to reduce chances of transmitting the infection to the baby. However, given numerous orphans, one can still be a parent by adopting or fostering.

Prayer

Leader: The Creator God, thank you for marriages;

All: Thank you God for giving us the responsibility to care for creation and for each other.

Leader: Thank you for marriages to honor your name;

All: Thank you for reminding us that it is possible to protect each other from HIV. We promise to obey you God;

All: We promise to be responsible partners and to speak openly about HIV/AIDS to our partners and to our children. Thank you for teaching us the truth.

Leader: Thank you because the truth will set us free

Benediction

May you remain one, as the Father, the Son and the Holy Spirit are One.

Closing song (Chichewa)

Chorus

Mau ali muntima mwanga // (God's message is in my heart)

kuti yesu ndi Mbuye // (That Jesus is the Christ)

Ndimtima ndikhulupilira // (In my heart I believe)

kuti anaukanso // (He rose again)

Ndimkamwa mwanga ndibvomereza // (With my mouth I confess)

Kuti Yesu ndi Mbuye // (That Jesus is the Christ)

Ndi mtima ndikhulupilira // (With my heart I believe)

Kuti Yesu ndi Mbuye // (that He is the Christ)

Ndipo anaukanso // (and he rose again)

(A Malawian Community Song)

Objects/symbols/ideas: Flowers, candles, testimonies: from HIV positive couples; old couples, photographs of happy couples, a basket of corn, drums and other musical instruments to go with the song.

By Isabel Apawo Phiri

4. Anniversary

Sermon Text: Exodus 12:1-14

Song

Njalo Njalo // (Always) 4x
Siyathandaza // (We pray)
Siyanikela // (We give)
Siyadumisa // (We praise)
Thina njalo // (Us always)
(Popular South African Chorus)

Introduction

An anniversary is the commemoration of a day when an important event took place in one's life. This can be a wedding anniversary or a day when one obtained promotion at work, or the day a loved one went to be with the Lord, or a day when one graduated from high school/college/ university. It is up to the individual to decide whether to celebrate such an occasion or not.

In relation to a marriage contract, an anniversary comes every year when a couple remembers the day they were joined together in holy matrimony. A marriage can also be taken as a commemoration ceremony; we can put it in line with the Passover. When two people come together in marriage, there are some wedding vows to be pronounced and these vows serve as a commitment to each other and to God. The time of the anniversary, is the time for a couple to revisit these vows.

In this age of HIV/AIDS, it is important for the couple to keep reminding each other of the promises they made before God. During the time of the Israelites, their enemy was the Egyptians, today the enemy of most marriages is HIV/AIDS, which has destroyed thousands of marriages due to marital unfaithfulness.

We Listen to the Word of God

This passage marks the end of the bondage of the Hebrew people by the Egyptians. The Passover was an annual event, which was instituted by the Hebrews to commemorate the end of their bondage. In this passage, certain rules are laid down on how this important event is to be celebrated. Every anniversary has its own celebration methods.

DETAILS OF THE TEXT
Verses 2:
> ➢ "This month…the first month"; this verse marks the beginning of the religious calendar of the people of Israel.

Verse 3:
> ➢ "The community of Israel" refers to all the people of Israel. They were to be gathered together to hear the instructions.

Verse 4:
> ➤ "At twilight," the ceremony was to start at a particular time.

Verse 7:
> ➤ "The blood" which was smeared on the door posts of all the houses of the people of Israel was to symbolize that a sacrifice was made to spare the life of the Israelites.

Verse 8:
> ➤ "The bitter herbs" were eaten as a reminder to the people of Israel of their experience in Egypt. "Bread without yeast" was a reminder that they ate in haste, and "roasted meat" was a reminder of their lives as shepherds.

Verse 11:
> ➤ "Passover" meant the Lord would pass over the houses of the Israelites when the angel of death came to kill the first born of the Egyptians.

Verse 14:
> ➤ "Celebrate it," is a celebration of the Lord's goodness to the people of Israel. This is still done among the Jews, even in our generation.

We Apply the Word of God to Ourselves

WHAT CAN WE LEARN?
- We need to take time to celebrate life.
- Marriage is an example of an event in one's life that can be celebrated every year. The time of the anniversary, is time for a couple to revisit their vows and celebrate the goodness of God in their lives.
- The presence of HIV/AIDS makes it even more important to celebrate each other's lives, e.g. birthdays and anniversaries.

WHAT DO WE HAVE TO CONFESS?
- Do we renew our marriage vows to God and to each other during wedding anniversaries?
- The blood of the lamb was used as a protection for the Israelites. Can the blood of Jesus be used to cleanse us from sin?
- In the case of the couple contracting HIV while already married, is it possible for that couple to use the anniversary as a reconciliation time?

WHAT CAN WE BE THANKFUL FOR?
- Despite the problems that people face in life, God has given us the opportunity to celebrate personal and community anniversaries.

WHAT CAN WE PRAY FOR?
- That we use occasions like anniversaries to mend broken relationships by remembering the original vows and promises.
- That God should help us to honor promises that we make.

We Apply the Word of God to the Congregation

WHAT CAN WE FEEL?
- Happy because God has given us occasions when we can remember the past events through communal celebrations.
- Sorry that we have not used these occasions to mend broken relationships.
- Sorry that we have forgotten the anniversaries of our loved ones and therefore given the impression that we do not care.

WHAT CAN WE BE?
- People who take time to remember other people's anniversaries.
- A community that uses anniversaries as an occasion to mend broken relationships and move on in happiness.
- A community that celebrates life.

WHAT CAN WE DO?
- Keep a diary of important events in our families and in our church community.
- Participate in the celebration of other people's events in our community.
- Special attention should be paid to celebrate events of the people who are HIV positive.

Conclusion: A Word on Society

A marriage is a covenant before God and couples should realize that when they make vows during the wedding, they are also doing it before God. If there is any unfaithfulness in the marriage, the couple should use events such as wedding anniversaries to renew their relationship with openness and love. In our society, we should take time to organize celebrations for anniversaries for people who are not able to organize for themselves, for example, anniversaries of people who are sick, poor or too old.

Prayer

Leader: Thank you God because you are the giver and protector of life;
All: Help us to do our part in the protection of life;
Leader: You have shown us how to celebrate events in life;
All: Empower us to want to participate and enjoy celebrations of ourselves, our loved ones and members of our community;
Leader: You are the light of the world.
All: Use us to bring your light to people who are not able to enjoy celebrations because of sickness, old age and poverty.

Song (Chichewa)
Nditzakutamandani Mulungu wanga // (I will praise you my God) (X2)
Mwachita zazikulu pamoyo wanga // (You have done great things in my life)
Ndidzakutamandani Mulungu wanga // (I will praise you my God)

Benediction

May you always experience the presence of God in your life. May you be strong in the face of adversaries. May you overcome the obstacles of life.

Objects/symbols/ideas: Food, flowers, candles, stories of people who celebrated anniversaries and what that mean to them, pictures from the original day, musical instruments.

By Isabel Apawo Phiri

5. Closing and Graduation Ceremony

Jeremiah 2:17

Instructions: The day before the ending of the workshop, ask the participants to write three to five lines of a commitment on implementing their training. This will be read aloud in the closing ceremony/worship. Prepare certificates of attendance for all of them and a Stoll for their ordination to serve. If you do not have certificates or Stolls, collect pebbles and give to each of them as symbols of the knowledge they received and which they must use and multiply. You may choose to use other relevant or available symbols for your context, audience or denominational background. Then assign different readers the lead parts of the service.

Introduction

With the HIV/AIDS epidemic, the church and society in general, are challenged to new learning and training, to undertake prevention, provision of quality care, and mitigating the impact of HIV/AIDS. Holding training, informative, skill-imparting, activist and advocate's workshops is a common and necessary reality. Raising funds and running such workshops is expensive and a serious service of *training soldiers of life* to undertake the war against HIV/AIDS. The need for commitment from those who attend the trainings to implement what they learned, is critical. Yet in the HIV/AIDS fight, we know that knowledge and education alone are not enough to mold people. We also need to appeal to their hearts and relationship with God, to see their training as God's call to serve God's people. This service is therefore prepared for closing and graduation worship/ceremony, marking the end of the workshop, and the beginning of service in ommunities. It may also be used for general graduation with diplomas, degrees and masters of ministers.

Call to Commitment

Leader 1:   Then the Lord said:
I have seen the misery of my people,
I have heard their cry,
I know their sufferings. (Exodus 3:7-8)

Leader 2:   Then I heard the voice of the Lord saying,
Whom shall I send, and who will go for us? (Isaiah 6:8)

Leader 3:   My People are destroyed because of lack of knowledge. (Hosea 4:6)

All:	Here am I; send me, (Isaiah 6:8) Until justice rolls down like waters, And righteousness like an ever-flowing stream. (Amos 5:24) Send us Lord.

Song

Thuma mina (2x) Thuma mina Somandla.
Send me Jesus (2x) Send me Jesus, I will go
(Thuma Mina, 166)

Leader 4:	What does the Lord require of you?
All:	To do justice, to love kindness, And to walk humbly with your God. (Micah 6:8)

Reading the Scripture Nehemiah 2:17

"You see the trouble we are in: Jerusalem lies in ruins, and its gates have been burned with fire. Come, let us rebuild the wall of Jerusalem, and we will no longer be in disgrace."

Granduants: *Read their commitment*

ALL:	We can make a difference in the HIV/AIDS struggle; Help us Lord to become your healing hands, in your hurting world.

Closing Song

We are walking in the light of God
(Thuma Mina, 166)

Sending Prayer

Leader 5:	Then I heard the voice of the Lord saying, Whom shall I send, and who will go for us? (Isaiah 6: 8)
Leader 6:	My people are destroyed because of lack of knowledge. (Hosea 4:6)
All:	Send us Lord, to be committed soldiers in the HIV/AIDS struggle; Until HIV/AIDS is reduced and eradicated, send us Lord; Until HIV/AIDS stigma and discrimination is eradicated, send us Lord; Until quality care is given to all AIDS suffers, send us Lord; Until all orphans & widows are protected, send us Lord. Until our hearts, souls and minds are healed, send us Lord.

Silence
All briefly reflect on their commitment.

Leader: You are my servant,
I have chosen you and not cast you off.
Do not fear, for I am with you,
Do not be afraid, for I am your God.
I will strengthen you,
I will help you,
I will uphold you with my victorious right hand. (Isaiah 41:9-11)

ALL: The Spirit of the Lord is upon us, for he has anointed us to preach the good news to the poor. He has sent us to proclaim freedom for the captives and recovery of sight for the blind, to release the oppressed, to proclaim the year of the Lord (Luke 4:18-19).

By Musa W. Dube

6. Death and Funerals

FUNERAL
Sermon Text: Luke 7:11-17

Introduction

To the leader: The congregation needs to be told that this sermon is not a judgment on the deceased, but an opportunity to teach about HIV/AIDS. This does not mean that the person has died of AIDS. Where possible this should be preached at a funeral of a person who has not died of AIDS, and the family should be consulted before hand to avoid misunderstanding. In short given the stigma it must be handed diplomatically

Prayer

Leader: God Almighty the Alpha and Omega, the beginning and the finisher of our lives, we come to you to celebrate life after death. We celebrate your example of compassion for those who are grieved. Thank you for reminding us that death does not have the last word. We acknowledge the comfort we receive from the message about the resurrection power. We thank you for the life of this person *(mention the name).*

All: Lord in your mercy, hear our prayer;

Leader: We thank you for all those people who make themselves available to take care of this person.

All: Lord in your mercy hear our prayer and let our cry come to you.

31

Song (Zulu/Ndebele)

Thula Sizwe // (Be still O Nation)
Ungabokhala // (Don't cry)
Ujehova wakho Uzokunqobe // (Jehova will conquer for you)
Inkuleko // (freedom)
Uzoyithola // (will be yours)
Ujehova wakho // (Your Jehova)
Uzokunqobela // (Will conquer for you)
        (Popular Southern African Song)

In today's African communities, funerals have become a common occurrence because of high mortality rates due to an increase in crime, the HIV/AIDS epidemic, poverty, wars, etc. Funerals are also occasions for much suffering because of accusations about witchcraft. Even when a person dies of AIDS, someone is accused of witchcraft. Most of the people who are accused of witchcraft are women. This is based on the African belief that death does not just happen. One's enemies cause it.

Suffering is worsened for the bereaved family when people know that the deceased has died of AIDS. This is because many people lack knowledge and therefore still associate AIDS with sin and stigma, even in Christian circles. Funerals in the urban areas have brought another side of suffering as they tend to be expensive. The relatives are pressured to show how much they care by having an expensive coffin and a big feast after the burial. AIDS sufferers are neglected when alive. Due to feelings of guilt, family members overspend on expensive coffins to cleanse themselves. This is also associated with our African belief that it is important to send a dead person off very well. This cultural belief is now being expressed through expensive funerals.

We Listen to the Word of God

Read the text of Luke 7:11-17

In the reading, Jesus raised a dead man because he had compassion for the widow, the dead person's mother.

DETAILS OF THE TEXT
➢ The man who died was an only child of a widow. According to Jewish tradition, this means that the woman had no male protection and was therefore at the bottom of the economic ladder.

➢ Jesus performed a miracle by raising the dead person. He did it because he had compassion on the woman. This should be taken as a sign, because we know that not everyone who died and came in contact with Jesus was raised. The fact that Jesus does not raise our dead relatives, does not mean that he has no compassion over us.

➢ Jesus raised the hopes of all the people who attended the funeral. Therefore, resurrection should be understood also in a wider sense, of restoring hope to the living.

We Apply the Word of God to Ourselves

WHAT CAN WE LEARN?
- That God intervenes in human suffering;
- That we should have compassion towards those who are mourning, and help them in any way we can;
- That we should have special compassion for widows;
- That we need to meet the needs of those who are suffering, e.g. bringing hope to those who do not have it.

WHAT DO WE HAVE TO CONFESS?
- Do we have the compassion of Jesus to help those who are in need?
- Do we intervene when people are accused falsely of witchcraft?
- Have we stopped feeling compassion towards the bereaved because of the frequency of deaths in our communities?
- Is there lack of compassion in us due to our judgmental attitudes towards people who suffer and die of AIDS?

WHAT CAN WE BE THANKFUL FOR?
- The fact that God is with God's people both in sorrow and in happiness;
- That even if a person is not raised from death in this world, there is hope for resurrection in the next world;
- That resurrection also means restoration of hope among the living.

WHAT CAN WE PRAY FOR?
- God to help us to put into practice the spirit of compassion, especially towards people who are suffering, i.e. the bereaved, widows, orphans;
- God to help us to live in the resurrection power; having the idea that there is life after death, but also refusing to be hopeless in our lives.

We Apply the Word of God to the Congregation

WHAT CAN WE FEEL?
- Sorry that we have not shown compassion to people in our congregations who are suffering;
- Repentance that we let fear of HIV/AIDS leads us into stigma and hopelessness.

WHAT CAN WE BE?
- Christians who are the hands and feet of Jesus Christ. We need to reach out to those who are suffering.

WHAT CAN WE DO?
- Funerals are community events to be shared by the whole congregation;
- Start a ministry to bring relief to those who are suffering;
- Show acceptance towards those who are living with HIV/AIDS, and the members of their family who are nursing them.

Conclusion: A Word on Society

Jesus did not ask the widow for the cause of her son's death before showing compassion to her. Our ministry, as Christians, is to show compassion and not to be judgmental about what has killed a person. Whether the person has died of AIDS or not, is not an issue before God. It should not be an issue to us. Our call is to comfort the sick and the grieved.

Prayer

Leader: The church of God is called to serve;

All: We are the church of God to bring compassion to the suffering,

Leader: Jesus did not discriminate against people.

All: We will follow your footsteps Lord, by not showing discrimination against the sick, widows and orphans.

Leader: God is the source of our courage;

All: Give us the courage to do what is right in all circumstances.

Leader: Let us pray for the bereaved that God should use us to comfort them.

All: It is right and good for us to comfort the bereaved.

Leader: Let us pray for the caregivers, who work under difficult conditions;

All: Lord, use us to relieve them from their pain,

Leader: Thank you God, because you left us with your Holy Spirit and the Christian community to comfort us during difficult times.
In Jesus name,

All: Amen.

Closing song (Zulu)

Halleluyah Hosanah (4x)
Siyakudumisa // (We adore you) (3x)
Nkosi ya makosi // (Lord of Lords)
Akeko Ofanana naye // (There is no one like you) (3x)
Nkosi ya makosi // (Lord of Lords)
Sizasonwalbile kuwena // (We will rest in you) (3x)
Nkosi ya makosi // (Lord of lords).

(Popular South African Chorus)

Benediction

May the peace of God, that passes all understanding, the love of God and the fellowship of the Holy Spirit, be with us all.

Objects/symbols/ideas: Candles, flowers, water, playing drums.

By Isabel Apawo Phiri

DEATH/RESURECTION
Sermon Text: John 11:1-44

Introduction

At Kgolagano College of Theological Education where I work, we always begin the day by sharing in prayer. At the end of the prayers, we take a moment to share our news with each other. Although we are just a small staff of seven, there is always someone who shares with the others that a family member has passed away. It is as though we are playing rounds, taking turns to report the death of a cousin today, the next day somebody else reporting the death of an uncle and so on. Most of us in Africa experience death on a daily basis given the HIV/AIDS context of today. In some places there is a great shortage of land in our towns and cities because it is taken up by graveyards. There is death all around, it is in the air, it is as though one could touch it.

We Listen to the Word of God

DETAILS OF THE TEXT

➢ This is a long narrative about the death and resurrection of Lazarus. It might be a good idea for the preacher to find a quick and creative way of re-telling the story rather than just a straight reading. One way could be by the story-teller becoming Martha or Mary and sharing her grief and delight at what happened. This is bound to raise the attention and interest of the congregation.

➢ The narrative shows Jesus' love for his three friends; Lazarus, Mary and Martha. It also shows his refusal to come when he heard that Lazarus was sick in Bethany, his encounter with Martha, his statement that he is the resurrection and life, Martha's confession of faith and the presence of the mourners. All these features need to come out in the re-telling. It should not be assumed that this is a familiar story which the congregation already knows.

➢ In this narrative, Jesus does not remain calm and undisturbed by the reality of death. He is not like one who is detached from the messy business of living. He is deeply disturbed by death's devastation, its force and finality. Jesus weeps.

➢ The second thing to note is that Jesus is bringer of resurrection and life. Jesus instructs the baffled and unprepared onlookers, "Unbind him, and let him go" (v.44). And immediately Lazarus is loosed from the bonds of death, freed from the shackles of the past, and liberated into a new future!

We Apply the Word of God to Ourselves and the Congregation

Although death besets us from all angles, the power of the resurrection keeps us going. We live on because the resurrection not just a futuristic reality, but an experience here and now. Like Martha and Mary, we say our brothers and sisters loosened and unbound from fear, hopelessness, and physical pain (through ARV drugs).

WHAT CAN WE LEARN?
Illustrations:

- During the terrible floods of Mozambique in 1999/2000, a poignant occurrence took place. As the waters of death were rushing and sweeping away everything in its way, some people took refuge on the trees. Among these was an expectant mother. It is hard to imagine how it happened, but somehow she gave birth on a tree, and she and the baby were rescued. During that moment life defied death, and in the midst of death there was life.

- In the midst of the ravages and death of so many victims of HIV/AIDS in Africa, Christ still brings resurrection and life. There are still life-enhancing experiences of people who do everything to 'stay alive', who embrace people living with AIDS (like Jesus embraced his friends at Bethany), and who devote all their life to stopping the spread of AIDS. Through these people and their ministries Christ is saying, "Unbind them and let them go."

WHAT CAN WE CONFESS?
- Sometimes we succumb too easily to the powers of death around us;
- Our failure to 'unbind' the many who live in the shadow of death around us.

WHAT CAN WE BE THANKFUL FOR?
- The gospel of Jesus Christ which promises life beyond death;
- The experiences of 'resurrection' in many people in our communities;
- The ministry of many Christians which brings life to the spiritually and emotionally dead.

WHAT CAN WE PRAY FOR?
- God, lift the dark cloud of death that hovers over the continent of Africa;
- Listen to the wailing cries of the mothers and children of our land;
- Wipe away our tears and take from us the scorn of AIDS related deaths;
- Help us Lord for we pray in the name of Jesus Christ. Amen

Song

He is lord, He is Lord,
He is risen from the dead,
And he is Lord.
Every knee shall bow,
Every tongue confess,
That Christ is Lord.   (Anonymous)

Suggested idea/symbols: Get someone to be either Martha or Mary and get her to tell the story of how Jesus came to raise Lazarus. Whoever does the re-telling could also try and contextualize, so that it becomes more meaningful for today.

By Moiseraela P. Dibeela

THREATS OF DEATH
Sermon Text: Luke 8:22-25

Introduction

"Little things that run and fail, and die in silence and despair." So run the lines of a poem I leaned in primary school. I still remember it because it reminds me of the precariousness and vulnerability of life. There are many things that threaten our lives in Africa today. Malaria is a major killer, HIV/AIDS and its opportunistic diseases, wars, road accidents, famine, floods the list goes on. Human existence is caught up in various storms of life and life is threatened on many fronts. Here our concern is with the scourge of HIV/AIDS. Who is there to calm this storm for us?

Reading the Word

Put these questions to the text:

Why do you think this happened to Jesus?
Who initiated this trip across the lake?
What happened to Jesus immediately after they set sail?
What happened to the boat?
What did the disciples do?
What do you think the disciples expected Jesus to do?
What did Jesus mean by the question, "Where is your faith?"
What does the question that the disciples asked in return, "Who is this?" tell us about their knowledge of Jesus?

Applying the Word of God to Ourselves

This story comes within a series of stories about the activities of Jesus as he goes about doing good. It is the miracle of stilling the storm. Those who live near lakes or oceans know how treacherous water can be. Even rivers in flood times are an awesome sight to behold. At its widest point Lake Malawi is about 80km. We were once caught in a storm. There were literally thousands of hills of water foaming at the crest, as the boat kept cutting through them as it sailed, moving up and down. Passengers reeled from side to side, as many kept vomiting. It was both an awful and awesome sight. Can you imagine someone sleeping through such a storm? Jesus actually did and he had to be woken up. He simply rebuked the storm and calm was restored.

This was a miracle, but what is a miracle? Usually, it is defined as an event contrary to the operation of the laws of nature. God and Godly people are capable of such fits, it is believed. Miracles are sometimes seen as a suspension of natural laws. Since nothing is impossible with God, God performs miracles all the time for His own glory. However, it may also be said that miracles happen when creative forces operate on a deeper or higher level, than what we are naturally accustomed, to as per the natural laws that we know. This means that healing is possible. Jesus speaks and reveals himself to us through his activity.

Go through these questions with the congregation:

- What does it mean to be a disciple of Jesus?
- Share a story of being caught in a storm on the lake or ocean?
- Suppose this was a parable, what are events in your life which could be likened to a storm?
- If you were one of the disciples would you have responded differently?
  Give reasons for your answer.
- What should our faith in Jesus mean for our lives? Share experiences in which God spoke or was revealed to you in some activity, or left you wondering who God is.

WHAT CAN WE LEARN?
- Threats to life can come suddenly from anywhere. The storm came suddenly upon them;
- Tiredness is inevitable after hard work, and rest is necessary;
- Solidarity is important in time of crisis;
- We can rely on Jesus to intervene;
- Faith in the ability of God to avert threats to life is necessary.

WHAT CAN WE CONFESS?
- Our lack of faith;
- Making Jesus the last resort;
- Allowing ourselves to fear.

WHAT CAN WE BE THANKFUL FOR?
- The presence of Jesus on our faith journey. He draws near, as on the road to Emmaus;
- The ability of Jesus to calm our storms;
- That we are not alone. God is always with us.

WHAT CAN WE PRAY FOR?
- The ability to recognize threats to life, and to deal with them effectively;
- The ability to overcome our fears, so as to trust more.

WHAT CAN WE FEEL?
- Fear;
- Surprise;
- Amazement;
- Wonder mixed with doubt.

WHAT CAN WE BE?
- People of faith;
- People of courage.

WHAT CAN WE DO?
- Turn to Jesus for help;
- Find more about who Jesus is;
- Assure the sufferer that HIV/AIDS is manageable death is postponable.

Song

When peace like a river
Attendeth my way,
When sorrows like sea billows roll;
Whatever my lot, Thou hast taught me to say,
It is well, it is well, with my Life!

It is well with my Life!

It is well, it is well, with my Life!

Though Satan should buffet,
Though trials should come;
Let this blessed assurance control,
That Christ has regarded my helpless estate,
And has shed his own blood for my Life.   (Hymns for Malawi, 158)

Prayer

Master, master, we are dying.
Don't you see the plague
That has engulfed entire peoples,
The HIV/AIDS plague,
A plague without a cure,
A plague so devastating.
Master, master, hear the Statistics:
Ten percent to thirty percent,
We are being wiped out.
Whole people and whole nations.
Have mercy on us, O loving Master.
Take pity upon the sheep of your fold.
Grant us life, grant us hope, grant us a cure.
Through the risen Lord, we beseech you.
                    Amen

Suggested Objects/symbols/ideas: Toy boat, water, pillow, oar or any other appropriate object.

By Augustine C. Musopule

7. Services for Tomb Unveiling

TOMB UNVEILING
Sermon Text: I Corinthians 15:35-58

Introduction

Due to the high rate of HIV/AIDS prevailing in sub-Saharan Africa, rituals associated with death are being performed with increased frequency. Tomb unveiling is a ritual in which the community seeks to remember the deceased, and to beautify his or her place of rest. HIV/AIDS has led to the need for more reflections on the religious significance of this ritual. Emphasis should be placed on its memorial character, as a celebration of the hope that the deceased will resurrect, as well as the need to fight HIV/AIDS stigma. Such Christian themes should minimize the concerns that tomb unveiling is steeped in traditional African culture.

Tomb unveiling provides an opportunity for the community to avoid HIV/AIDS stigma and to recognize the devastation brought by the epidemic. It is a reminder of the pain of death, but it also points to the regeneration of the living. The ritual is a foreshadowing of the resurrection and should draw attention to the beginning of a new life for both the deceased and the living. It should also reflect the thanksgiving dimension and articulate a sense of hope.

We Listen to the Word of God

Skeptics consider death as final. Some philosophers, poets, singers and others have portrayed the grave as decisive. However, the Christian faith is built on the conviction that Christ has been raised from the dead, being the first fruits of those who have fallen asleep (I Corinthians 15:20). In the situation of HIV/AIDS, it is necessary to develop a theology of hope and life. How the community of the faithful needs to be resurrected from its hopelessness and despair, should receive special emphasis.

DETAILS OF THE TEXT
Verse 36:
➤ Death is a precondition for life. As we get depressed by the reality of so much death, disease and poverty around us, let us be empowered by the knowledge that what is sown does not come to life unless it dies. However, we should acknowledge that most deaths due to HIV/AIDS are in fact preventable and postponable.

Verses 42-44:
➤ The transformation from a physical to a spiritual body is the underlying theme of resurrection. Though our bodies are subject to processes of disintegration while in the flesh, the spiritual body is imperishable. Tomb unveiling is undertaken as a celebration of hope that the deceased will put on this new spiritual body. It anticipates the immortality of the deceased. Please note that the resurrection also applies to the living, in that they need to overcome the fear caused by HIV/AIDS in order to lead wholesome lives. African holism challenges body/spirit dichotomy and the body should not be devalued.

Verses 51-55:

➢ The last trumpet is a significant Christian eschatological symbol. It captures vividly the ushering in of the kingdom of God on earth. The dead will be raised imperishable and the sting of death shall be no more. Jesus Christ, who himself defeated death, avails victory to those who have faith. Tomb unveiling is a foretaste of this mystery to be unveiled. The tomb where the deceased is sleeping is but a temporary dwelling place: upon the sound of the trumpet they shall join those who put on immortality. Life will finally triumph over death. Despite the reality of HIV/AIDS, we need this restoration of hope.

We Apply the Word of God to Ourselves and the Congregation

WHAT CAN WE LEARN?
- Death is not the end of existence;
- Tomb unveiling is a celebration of life;
- We need to consider the living as undergoing the resurrection, in terms of their sense of hope.

WHAT DO WE HAVE TO CONFESS?
- Our failure to act in the light of preventable deaths in our HIV/AIDS contexts;
- Our tendency to attribute all deaths to God's will;
- Our complacency with forces of death, poverty, violence and corrupt government;
- We spend too much money on funerals and not enough on saving life.

WHAT CAN WE BE THANKFUL FOR?
- The time that the deceased had with us;
- Medical efforts in fighting HIV/AIDS;
- The promise and hope of resurrection.

WHAT CAN WE PRAY FOR?
- That God gives us the strength to continue working for positive change in the struggle against HIV/AIDS. We also require wisdom to use occasions like tomb unveiling to communicate messages of hope.

We Apply the Word of God to the Congregation

- Ask members what tomb unveiling means to them.
- Does tomb unveiling remind them of the realities of HIV/AIDS?
- What is the congregation prepared to do to fight forces of death?

Conclusion: A Word on Society

Tomb unveiling should not become a financial burden on society. Instead, it should galvanize leaders at various levels to actively contribute to the fight against HIV/AIDS. As memorial stones are erected for the deceased, society should be challenged to pause and formulate strategies that promote life.

Song

Hosanna (x2)
Tichandoimba Hosanna
Tichitenderera pachigaro chaMambo
Tichandoimba Hosanna
Hosanna (2x)
We shall sing hosanna
As we circle the Lord's throne
We shall sing hosanna

(Popular chorus, author unknown)

Re tla bina hosanna (3x)
Re dikologa sitilo sa kgosi
Re tla bina hosanna

(Anonymous)

Prayer

God of all nations,
Lord of life, we thank you for our Lord, Jesus Christ.
We praise you for the gift of life;
We rejoice at your promise of resurrection;
We acknowledge your victory over death.
Grant us the courage to challenge
Systems of death and misery.
Hear us and help us,
As we search for abundant life,
Now and forever.
Forgive our sins,
Through Jesus Christ. Amen

Suggested Objects/Symbols/ideas: White or black cloth (purity, life, peace); grain (life, potentiality); stone (permanence, beauty).

By Ezra Chitando

8. A Healing and Memorial Service

Sermon Text: Psalm 23

Instructions: This memorial service is designed for small groups such as Sunday school classes, workshops, conferences, women's and youth meetings. It seeks to heal the participants, as well as to help everyone acknowledge that HIV/AIDS is close to all of us; that we are all affected. It also helps to break the silence and the stigma. It also seeks to deal with hopelessness by underlining that God is with us; God's light is still shining upon our situation.

Call to Worship

Leader:	We are your world and your people;
All:	You created us with your hands;
Leader:	We are made in your likeness;
All:	You created us in your image;
Leader:	We are people of your love;
All:	You created us and you created us good.

Song

Oh Lord my God, when I in awesome wonder,
Consider all the works thy hands have made.
I see the stars, I hear the roaring thunder,
Thy power throughout the universe displayed.
    Then sings my soul, my savior God to thee,
    How great thou art, how great thou art,(2x)
And when I think, that God his son not sparing,
Sent him to die, I scarce can take it in.
That on the cross, my burden gladly bearing,
He bled and died, to take away my sin
    Then sings my soul...

Confession

Leader:	Today your world is infected and by HIV/AIDS;
All:	We are infected and affected by HIV/AIDS.
Leader:	Today Life is under threat;
All:	Many of us are already sick and hopeless.
Leader:	Today we are also suffering from HIV/AIDS stigma;
All:	Many of us have been judgmental.
All:	We confess our ignorance, fears and confusions;
	We confess our judgmental attitude;
	We confess our failure to love and accept.
	Help us to see your face in the faces of.
	All who are infected and affected by HIV/AIDS.
	Help us to leave all judgment to You.
	Help us to be your healing hands in a hurting world.

Song

Thuma Mina (2x) Thuma mina Somandla
Send me Jesus (2x) Send me Jesus, I will go.

(Thuma Mina, No. 166)

Leader:	We are all affected by HIV/AIDS;
All:	We are the body of Christ.
Leader:	We have lost close relatives;
All:	Heal our bodies.
Leader:	We have lost close friends and neighbors;
All:	Heal our hearts.
Leader:	We have lost church and work mates;
All:	Heal our spirits.
Leader:	We have lost our hope;
All:	Heal our minds.
Leader:	We put our trust in you;
All:	You are Emmanuel,
	You are God With Us. (Matthew 1:23)
	You will never leave us or forsake us; (Hebrews 13:5)
	You will be with us to the end of ages. (Matthew 28:20)

ALL RECITE: Psalm 23:1-6

God is my shepherd, I shall not be in want.
God makes me lie down in green pastures,
God leads me beside still waters,
God restores my soul.
God leads me in the path of righteousness
For God's name's sake.
Even though I walk in the valley of the shadow of death,
I will fear no evil,
For you are with me,
Your rod and your staff,
They comfort me.
You prepare a table before me, in the presence of my enemies,
You anoint my head with oil,
My cup overflows.
Surely goodness and mercy shall follow me
All the days of my life,
And I shall dwell in the house of God for ever.

Song

We have a Shepherd *(You may choose another appropriate song)*

Re nale Modisa, re nale Modisa (2x) (We have a shepherd, we have a shepherd)

Morena orile ke modisa yo Molemo (The Lord said, he is the good shepherd)
Morena o rile ga a ketla a re tlogela (The Lord said, he will never leave us)
Morena o rile o nale rona ka metlha (The Lord said, will be with us forever)
Re nale Modisa (We have a shepherd)

Re nale Modisa, re nale Modisa (2x) (We have a shepherd, We have a shepherd)

Morena o rile ke Modisa wa rona (The Lord said, he is the good shepherd)
Morena o rile ga re ketla re tlhako sepe (The Lord we will never lack anything)
Morena o rile o tla refudisa mo mafolong a matalana (The Lord said he will lead us to green pastures)
Re nale Modisa (We have a shepherd)

Re nale Modisa, re nale Modisa (2x) (We have a shepherd, we have a shepherd)

Lefa dira di ka go dikaganyetsa (Even if enemies could surround you)
Lefa meleko e ka go tlhasela (Even if temptations could attack you)
Lefa o ka feta kgothong e lefifi (Even if you pass through the dark valley)
O nale Modisa (You have a shepherd)

Re nale Modisa, re nale Modisa (2x) (We have a shepherd, we have a shepherd)
(By Musa W. Dube)

The Main Candle is lit

Leader: This candle is lit to symbolize that God is with us, and God will always be with us. It is also lit in memory of those who have gone before us, who are awaiting resurrection. It is lit to break the silence and the stigma—to openly say we that have relatives and friends who have died of HIV/AIDS. It is above all, lit for our own healing, to rekindle our hope in Emmanuel, God With Us.

One person at a time stands up, goes to the table, lights a candle from the main candle, calls the name of a relative/friend/neighbors/workmate who has died of HIV/AIDS. The rest respond with the following:

ALL: Heal our land Oh Lord; bind our wounds.

Closing Song

Blessed assurance, Jesus is mine,
Oh what a foretaste, of glory divine.
Born of the Spirit, lost in his blood,
Heir of salvation, purchase of God.

45

Chorus:
This is my story, this is my song,
Praising my Savior, all the day long.

Perfect submission, perfect delight,
Visions of rapture, now burst in my sight.
Angels descending, bringing from above,
Echoes of mercies, and whispers of love.

Perfect submission, all is at rest,
I in my Savior, I am happy and blessed.
Watching and waiting, and looking above,
Filled with His goodness, and lost in His love.

Closing Prayer

Leader: We put our trust in you.
All: You are Emmanuel;
You are God with us. (Matthew 1:23)
You will never leave us or forsake us. (Hebrews 13:5)
You will be with us to the end of ages. (Matthew 28:20)
Amen

Objects/ideas/symbols: Candles, or you may choose to use any other objects that represent healing, God's unfailing presence and a memorial service.

By Musa W. Dube and Fulata L. Moyo

9. Thanksgiving

SERVICE ON THANKSGIVING
Sermon Text: I Chronicles 29:10-19

Prayer

O shout to the Lord in triumph, all earth:
Serve the Lord with gladness,
And come before his face with songs of joy.

Know that the Lord is God:
It is he who has made us and we are his;
We are his people and the sheep of his pasture.

Come into his gates with thanksgiving,
And into his courts with praise:
Give thanks to him, and bless his holy name.

For the Lord is good, his loving mercy is forever:
His faithfulness throughout all generations.
(Taken from Psalm 100)

Song

Tsohle Tsohle Di entswe Ke Wena. Modimo Re Boka Wena.
All things have been created by you Lord God. We thank and praise you.
(This is a popular chorus well known in several Southern African countries. An alternative thanksgiving song may be sung).

Introduction

Every Sunday should be a thanksgiving Sunday. Every service should be a thanksgiving service. Every day should be a thanksgiving day. This is so, because when we consider our situation carefully, we will realize the extent to which we are beneficiaries and dependants of God's grace. It is God's protection and providence that makes it possible for us to live from day to day. In recent times, nothing has made us realize our indebtedness to God more than the devastating advent of the HIV/AIDS epidemic. As we learn more and more about the disease, its extent and the manner in which it is spread and transmitted, we each realize that we all could be infected and we all are affected. HIV positive people are no more sinners than HIV negative people. HIV negative people are no more saintly than HIV positive people. We therefore need to thank God for HIV negative people, and to ask God to preserve them as such. Similarly and even more so, we need to thank God for HIV positive people. They are the faces of Jesus in our midst. In them, we see the hope that Jesus inspired in us. In them we see the broken body of Christ. They teach us about the beauty and preciousness of life. Many of them live life as a gift - one day at a time. In them, we see ourselves, truly as we are. Let us thank God for HIV positive people, for God alone can give them peace and healing.

We Listen to the Word of God

A pre-warned and pre-selected member of the congregation may be asked to read the powerful prayer of thanks by King David in Chronicles 29:10-19

DETAILS OF THE TEXT
- This moving *thanksgiving prayerful passage* - uttered through the mouth of David, the great king of Israel - is the prelude to the building of the Temple. It is a task that David reckoned he would carry out. But God forbade him because he is a warrior, and he has shed blood (Chronicles 28:3). Instead, God chose Solomon his son to carry out the task. David informs the people and Solomon about this command of God.

- People responded overwhelmingly in support of Solomon and in support of the temple building project. It is the enthusiastic and generous response of the people that inspired David to utter the beautiful words of thanks and praise found in Chronicles 29:10-19. It was an occasion to acknowledge the generosity of people, but above all, God's initial generosity, which makes it possible for people to be generous at all.

> There is something powerful about a person in authority recognizing a greater authority. "Yours, O Lord, is the greatness and the power and the glory and the majesty and the splendor, for everything in heaven and on earth is yours". Ordinarily, kings would assume, if not insist, that greatness, power, glory and majesty, rightfully belong to them and to no one else. Furthermore, King David is able to see through the fact that even when humans give to God, they do nothing special in that what they give to God, belongs to God anyway.

We Apply the Word of God to Ourselves

WHAT CAN WE LEARN?
- God and God alone deserves our thanksgiving.
- No one is exempt from giving thanks to God even those who appear to 'have it all' - HIV negative people have as much reason to be thankful for life as HIV positive people are.
- We must give back to God what belongs to God. Glory, authority, honour and majesty are God's property. God has copyright on these. It is important that even in these trying times of the HIV/AIDS pandemic, we give honour and thanks where they belong, namely to God.
- Calamities such as HIV/AIDS may cause people to shift loyalty from God to other gods. It may cause them to feel resentfulness instead of thanksgiving to God. From David, we learn that even when God prevents us from accomplishing our ambitions, we should nevertheless be thankful.

WHAT DO WE HAVE TO CONFESS?
- We often compete with God for praise and honour. Our churches can fall into this trap.
- We often overrate our gifts to God.
- In the face of HIV/AIDS, thanksgiving may be relegated to the backseat.
- We often take God's gifts for granted.

WHAT CAN WE BE THANKFUL FOR?
- HIV negative people;
- HIV positive people;
- Life, whether we are HIV positive or not;
- God's many gifts.

WHAT CAN WE PRAY FOR?
- Hope in the midst of pain and despair;
- HIV negative people to act in ways that will keep them negative;
- HIV positive people to have hope and appreciate life;
- HIV positive people to lead responsible life.

We Apply the Word of God to the Congregation

WHAT CAN WE FEEL?
- Thankful that God loves both HIV positive and negative people equally;
- Thankful for the gift of life;
- Hopeful for healing and restoration;
- Sorry that we are often resentful and bitter, instead of thankful.

WHAT CAN WE BE?
- Joyful, hopeful and thankful Christians in spite of the HIV/AIDS pandemic;
- Responsible HIV positive people;
- Responsible HIV negative people.

WHAT CAN WE DO?
- Lead thankful lives;
- Lead responsible lives as HIV negative people;
- Lead responsible lives as HIV positive people;
- Become ambassadors of hope.

Conclusion: A Word on Society

Even though our life ambitions (such as King David's ambition to build the temple) are no longer achievable due to the effects of HIV/AIDS, either on ourselves or on those whom we love, we must trust God to still 'get the job done'. The millions of African orphans who lost both parents because of HIV/AIDS, need to know that the job of bringing them up into responsible adulthood can still be done. If their parents could not build the temple, God can use them and their descendants to build it. The messages of doom and hopelessness around HIV/AIDS must be confronted with concrete and proactive Christian actions of hope and goodwill. In these, we as Christians must build alliances with other actors in society. Above all, we must maintain a posture of thanksgiving both for HIV negative and HIV positive people.

Prayer of Commitment
Lord Jesus Christ, in these times of death and hopelessness, we pledge our loyalty to you. You are our hope. In these times of anger and bitterness, we offer our thanksgiving to you. We commit ourselves to becoming ambassadors of hope. We undertake to witness for you with thanksgiving.

Song
Thank you Jesus Amen
(This song has the advantage that it can be sung in many different languages)

Benediction
We say together the 'Prayer for Africa'
God bless Africa,
Guard her peoples,
Guide her rulers,
And grant her peace. Amen

Symbols/Objects and Commitments: Testimonies from people who 'survived,' and HIV/AIDS tests - regardless of the results. A bowl of fruit or other forms of harvest.

By Tinyiko S. Maluleke

THANKSGIVING
Sermon Text: Revelations 2:1-7

Introduction

The message to the church in Ephesus, is part of the apocalypse of John. Written in the form of a popular drama, the book of Revelation is a sharp and critical commentary on the historical events of the first Century C.E. At this time the Church went through some of the most stern opposition and gruesome persecution. The church lost some of its leading figures, such as the apostles, its first deacons, and all who dared to speak against the tyranny of the time. All of them were tortured and killed for their loyalty to Christ Jesus.

This is the context within which the book of Revelation was written. Christians were living under Roman rule, and one of the expectations of this rule was that all Roman citizens were to worship the emperor. This would have been a gross violation of one of the basic tenets of the Christian faith. For the Christians, they professed that only Jesus is Lord! They would worship none other than the Nazarene who was crucified, buried in a borrowed grave, and on the third day, rose from the dead, triumphant over evil and death. This faith, and the expectation by Emperor Nero and his successors that all citizens must worship him, set the stage for a collision of worldviews. The book of Revelation, therefore, reflects in a dramatic way, the response of the people of God to the pressures of their time.

We Listen to the Word of God

DETAILS OF THE TEXT

➢ The letter to the church in Ephesus gives a positive appraisal of the Christian's witness there. In the midst of seismic events such as oppression, murders of Christians, emperor worship, and fear amongst many, Christians in Ephesus have something to celebrate:

> *I know your works, your toil and your patient endurance. I know that you cannot tolerate evildoers; you have tested those who claim to be apostles but are not, and have found them to be false."* (v. 2)

The text though does not just give a positive view of the Christians at Ephesus. It is also sharply critical of them and calls them to repentance:

> *But I have this against you; that you have abandoned the love that you had at first. Remember then from what you have fallen; repent, and do the works you did at first. (vv.4-5a)*

We Apply the Word of God to Ourselves and the Congregation

We need to ask ourselves what the spirit is saying to the Church in Africa today. Like the Spirit said to the Church in Ephesus, "I know your works," the Spirit also has some things to say to the Church in Africa today. What can we be commended for in relation to HIV/AIDS?

WHAT CAN WE CONFESS?
Perhaps the spirit is saying to us today:
- "I know your denial." This is what the spirit is saying to the Church today, for we still deny that the church too is ravaged by HIV/AIDS like everybody else.
- "I know the way you stigmatize my people," for the Church in Africa continues to ostracize those who are infected with the HIV/AIDS.
- "I know your complacency," for the Church in Africa continues to lag behind in the fight against the HIV/AIDS epidemic, especially the fight against poverty, gender inequalities and the abuse of children's rights and national corruption, all of which fuel the diseases.

WHAT CAN WE BE THANKFUL FOR?
Thanksgiving in Africa can be difficult, because it often seems that there is little to be thankful for. Many people in Sub-Saharan Africa continue to live in the shadow of death because of poverty and HIV/AIDS. A lot of us are depressed because our loved ones are sick, and many have lost hope. However, we should celebrate the tenacity of the African spirit in spite of these circumstances. Despite our troubles, many rise every morning to take their children to school, to nurse the sick, to feed the hungry, and to continue with life. Many find joy in songs of praise to God. For this energy, for the spirit that defies the problems that beset us – we must be thankful. Let us be thankful for:
- Christians and churches which are involved in home-based care ministry;
- Church projects including day care centers for orphans, awareness programmes and HIV/AIDS campaigns;
- Pastors who teach, bury the dead and comfort the mourners;
- Many other HIV/AIDS activists.

WHAT CAN WE PRAY FOR?
Prayer
When we go in the morning, you are there Lord, and when we wake up in the morning you are there watching over us. You look upon us like a hen caring for her young ones. When we ask, "Where is God?" You answer, "Can a mother forsake a child whom she bore?" Even if she were to do so, I would never abandon you! Thank you Lord for your promises to us. Thank you for sustaining us in the mist of our troubles.

As we celebrate our faith in you, and your works among us, we pray for your guidance in our ministry. We pray for your guidance so that we may not be just bystanders in the fight against HIV/AIDS. We pray that you may make us compassionate and loving to those who are affected and infected by HIV/AIDS. Amen!!

Song
Count your blessings, name them one by one

Suggested objects: The leader could bring a jar of water, a three legged pot and perhaps corn or grains - symbols of life for Africans. It may be useful to explain the significance of these in the service.

By Moiseraele P. Dibeela

ACÇÃO DE GRAÇAS
Texto Sugerido: I Crónicas 29:10-19

Introdução

Muitas igrejas celebram o dia de Acção de Graças pelo menos uma vez por ano. Dependendo da maneira como os líderes dessas igrejas ou paróquias preparam o envento, essa celebração pode ser caracterizada por muita euforia, louvores e dávidas, assim como pode não passar de uma celebração igual às que se fazem cada domingo. O rei David, ao liderar esta oração, ensina-nos que a líderança, seja ela política ou religiosa, desempenha um papel fundamental em todas as faces da vida de um povo.

Escutemos a Palavra de Deus

Leia o texto. Sublinhe com um lápis as palavras mais importantes.

DETALHE
VV. 10-18:
➢ David louva a Deus e faz entrega das ofertas que ele e o povo dedicaram à construção do Templo.
V.19:
➢ Entrega a Deus a orientação espiritual do seu filho Salomão.

A Palavra de Deus para nós.

QUE PODEMOS APRENDER?
• Que uma boa liderança, seja ela religiosa ou de outra natureza, é sempre muito importante.
• Que o povo está sempre pronto para seguir as orientações dos seus líderes.
• Que na era do HIV/SIDA, a palavra de Líderes, pode ser decisava para o seu cambate.

QUE TEMOS DE CONFESSAR?
• Que muitas vezes falta visão à nossa liderança.
• Que os nossos problemas ocupam todo o nosso tempo e não deixam espaço para uma Acção de Graças.
• Que muitos não dão a devida atenção aos problemas causados pelo HIV/SIDA.
• Que muitos não sabem distinguir o que é bom daquilo que é mau nas suas celebrações da sexualidade.

EM QUE DEVEMOS ESTAR GRATOS A DEUS?
- À misericórdia de Deus que nunca nos abandona.

QUE DEVEMOS PEDIR NAS NOSSAS ORAÇÔES?
- Q ue o Espírito Santo ilumine e oriente os nossos dirigentes a todos os níveis.
- Que todos sejamos capazes de dar Acção de Graças condignamente.
- Que toda a nossa vida seja guiada por Deus.

PREGAMOS A LEI DE DEUS

Os Provérbios no seu capítulo 22.6, dizem:« *Instrui ao menino no caminho em que deve andar; e até quando envelhecer, não se desviará dele*». Estas palavras sábias são uma advertência permanente. Muitas vezes lamentamos pela falta de bons resultados nas tarefas em que nos empenhamos. Pode ser que algumas vezes tenhamos razão, mas muitas vezes somos culpados (as). O nosso comportamento, as nossas atitudes, é o que fica gravado nas pessoas. Devemos, pois, preocuparmo-nos pela instrução correcta dos mais novos (as). O HIV/SIDA exige que a educação sexual seja feita na tenra idade. Que os (as) mais novos (as) aprendam a respeitar-se e a respeitar o próximo. Devem saber o que é bom e o que é prejudicial para a sua própria saúde e para a comunidade. A família cristã deve unir-se no combate contra as forças da morte e na proclamação do nome do seu salvador Jesus Cristo.

CANCAO

Escolha uma canção que esteja de acordo com o tema.

ORAÇÂO

Senhor, agradecemos-te por este dia tão especial. Aprendemos que todos os passos que damos na vida devem ter uma motivação e devem ser dedicados a ti. Aprendemos também que a sexualidade é um dos teus dons e deve ser praticado para o teu louvor e dignificação. Os (as) nossos filhos (as) merecem por isso, ser bem instruídos (as) para que o pratiquem de uma maneira mais correcta e saudável e humana.Faça com que saibam escolher o melhor. E que lutem para a erradicação do HIV SIDA no mundo. Perdoe, Senhor todo misericordioso, a nossa tendência de escutar os maus conselhos. Conduz os nossos passos nos caminhos que levem a ti. Pedimos isso tudo na confiança de que nos darás, em nome de Jesus Cristo. Amen

Objectos sugeridos: Uma peneira cheia de diferentes tipos de fruta.

Por: Felicidade N. Cherinda

Part 2
Services on the Church Calendar/Rituals/Events

1. Christmas
> Matthew 1:18-24 (Cheryl Dibeela)
> Lucas 1:26-38 (Felicidade N. Cherinda)

2. Baptism
> Mark 1:9-11 (Augustine C. Musopule)

3. Lord's Supper
> I Corinthians 11:23-24 (Tinyiko S. Maluleke)
> Lucas 22:14-23 (Felicidade N. Cherinda)

4. Good Friday and Easter
> Mark 15:16-41 (Moiseraele P. Dibeela)

5. Resurrection/Restoration
> Luke 24:1 (Canon Gideon Byamugisha)
> Mark 16:1-8 (Ezra Chitando)

6. Ascension
> Luke 24:50-53 (Musa W. Dube)

7. World AIDS Day
> Isaiah 65:17-23 (Canon Gideon Byamugisha)

1. Christmas

CHRISTMAS AND FATHERHOOD
Sermon Text: Matthew 1:18-24

Introduction

Current research records indicate that females head 47% of the households in Botswana. This figure does not include the number of teenage mothers who bring up children without the support of the fathers. The theme of fatherhood therefore, seems to me to be an appropriate one to address. Single motherhood has become a common feature, and acceptable within many African societies. Single mothers are often left to take responsibility for their children in the absence of the fathers. This has left women more vulnerable than usual. Most of these women live under the poverty datum line. The children in such families are open to conditions of malnutrition, juvenile delinquency, crime, etc. The women themselves are exposed to exploitation, as they often have no choice but to opt for favors in return for money, or sometimes have to endure abusive relationships for the sake of the financial benefits. Survival becomes the main concern for these women. Even the laws and policies do not protect women, as they do not take seriously the responsibility that fathers ought to have for their children. This is especially so in respect to the laws and benefits of child maintenance. These are all contributing factors, and have worsened the HIV/AIDS epidemic.

We listen to the Word of God

DETAILS OF THE TEXT

Unlike the other gospels that seem to downplay the role of Joseph in the birth of Jesus, Matthew focuses on him. Here we learn that he was engaged to Mary when he discovered that she was pregnant. Joseph was filled with a lot of doubt as to whether he should divorce her, however after some divine intervention, he eventually decides to keep the matter quiet and marry Mary. I believe he did not do this only to protect her from the rejection and discrimination of society, but also because his conscious could not allow him to leave Mary on her own to take care of the child. Joseph never left Mary's side in the raising of their children.

We Apply the Word of God to Ourselves

WHAT CAN WE LEARN?
- That fatherhood is important to the development of children;
- That single mothers need a lot of support and encouragement;
- That fatherhood needs prayer and God's divine intervention.

WHAT DO WE HAVE TO CONFESS?
- That we often down play the role of fathers in bringing up and nurturing children;
- That lack of fatherhood has contributed to HIV/AIDS spread.

WHAT CAN WE BE THANKFUL FOR?
- For all the fathers that dutifully and lovingly look after their children;
- For single mothers, who in spite of the harsh living conditions, take care and provide for their children;
- That God is the father of all;
- That God is the parent of all the orphans.

WHAT CAN WE PRAY FOR?
- The many women who endure abusive relationships because they are financially dependent and need the money to support their families;
- Fathers who do not support their partners in raising the children;
- Child-headed homes of orphans.

We Apply the Word of God to our Church and Society

WHAT CAN WE DO?
- Teach about gender and HIV/AIDS, especially in relation to fatherhood;
- Become advocates for the equality and equal responsibility of women and men;
- Take care of orphans.

Song

The leader may choose any appropriate song.

Prayer

God our father of all-humankind,
You have not fallen short in your role as the father, ever.
You love, you take care, and you gently guide us.
Oh God, we need your guidance for fatherhood in Africa,
Guidance to take care and love those whom they have brought into this world.
We pray for all those people, who have not yet felt the love of a father in their lives. We pray for those who only know violence and abuse; those whose lives are empty and full of hurt. Guide us Father, as you guided Joseph. Amen

Suggested Symbols/ ideas: Artwork and sculptures around family.

By Cheryl Dibeela

NATAL
Texto Sugerido: Lucas 1:26-38

Oração

Graças te damos, Senhor todo poderoso, pelo anúncio de vida, que enche os nossos corações de alegria e de esperança. Hoje em dia, muitas mulheres nascem filhos doentes e condenados à morte certa. O HIV/SIDA transformou momentos de alegria em terror. Quem outro poderá salvar-nos senão tu? Sabemos que apesar da presença desta terrível doença entyre nós continuas a amar-nos. Por isso já é possível uma mãe infectada nascer uma criança saudável. Obrigada Senhor. Temos a certeza de que mais cedo do que possamos imaginar, medicamentos para a cura, serão descobertos. Dá-nos Senhor a graça de ver esses dias, pelo amor de Teu Filho, Jesus Cristo. Amen

Canção
Escolher uma canção de Natal

Vamos Escutar a Palvra de Deus

Leia o texto e sublinhe com um lápis as palavras mais importantes.

DETALHES
VV. 26-27:
➢ Introduzem-nos as personagens envolvidas, o lugar e o tempo em que o acontecimento teve lugar.

VV. 28-29:
➢ Dá-nos a conhecer o tipo de saudação que modificou a vida de Maria.

VV. 30-37:
➢ A natureza do Filho a nascer e a promessa da presença constante do Espírito Santo na vida de Maria.

V 38:
➢ Maria aceita o desafio com humildade.

Introdução

O Evangelho de Lucas é o único que nos conta com pormenor a história do nascimento de Jesus. Chama a nossa atenção para uma mulher até então desconhecida. Maria, mulher de fé, aceitou ficar grávida desafiando desse modo a tradição, a religião, a cultura e pôs em perigo relacções familiares. O Natal é um evento que nos lembra o Nascimento de Cristo, é um momento da história da salvação do mundo. Na luta contra o HIV/SIDA é preciso enfrentar e desafiar tudo e todos. Desde crenças, usos e costumes, e doutrina da igreja. A fé em Deus e a presença permanente do Espírito Santo,vão ajudar para a transformação de mentalidades e fazer com que a luta não seja em vão.

Palvra de Deus para nós.

QUE PODEMOS APRENDER?
- Que a eleição divina está sempre presente e continua a surpreender-nos;
- Que essa eleição não distingue as pessoas através da idade, sexo, condição social ou cor da pele;
- Que o Espírito Santo age em nós e nos orienta na tomada de decisões;
- Que devemos encarar positivamente os desafios que nos são colocados pelo HIV/SIDA;
- Que escutar a Palavra de Deus, é aceitar ir fazer o trabalho, seja ele qual for.

QUE TEMOS DE CONFESSAR?
- Que nos falta fé para encarar o desconhecido com coragem;
- Que os tabus e o egoísmo impedem-nos de agir no momento certo;
- Que às vezes as coisas acontecem sem o nosso control;
- Que o Natal tornou-se momento de festas e não de celebração da vida;
- Que o Natal, às vezes torna-se momento de divórcio e de suicídio, porque alguns não conseguem dar prendas e outros (as) não se conformam com o abandono.

QUE TEMOS DE AGRADECER?
- Conhecimento que Deus tem de nós;
- Convite que nos endereça para o servir;
- A proteção incondicional do Espírito Santo à nossa vida;
- Deus que se torna homem para nos salvar;
- Interesse de Deus pelo mundo;
- Para Deus nada é impossível.

Palavra de Deus para a Sociedade

QUE DEVEMOS PEDIR NA NOSSA ORAÇÂO?
- Para a igreja ser firme na proclamação da salvação na era do HIV/SIDA;
- Para Deus inspirar toda a gente e em especial a mulher, na luta contra o HIV/SIDA;
- Que nos ensine a amar os nossos filhos mesmo antes do seu nascimento.

Objectos: Desenho, fotografia ou escultura de uma mulher com um bebé nas costas.

Por: Felicidade N. Cherinda

2. Baptism

Sermon Text: Mark 1:9-11

Introduction

In order to appreciate this text, it will be important to put it in its proper context. Mark 1:1 gives us that context. Remember that Mark is writing this gospel many years after the events he is reporting. Therefore, the beginning that he is referring to is not simply the story of John the Baptist and Jesus' baptism, but rather the entire gospel. Jesus' humanity was not in doubt, but rather his divinity. Therefore, it was imperative for Mark to begin with a divine affirmation of who Jesus was. Jesus was not Son of God by adoption or simply anointment, but rather by being genuinely so.

We Listen to the Word of God

Verse 9:
➤ Baptism can mean different things to different people: ritual cleansing, the washing of sins, dying to sin and rising in newness of life, and so forth. For Jesus, it meant identifying himself with the mission of John the Baptist, and with sinners; and he finds in this an opportunity to be inaugurated into his own ministry for sinners.

Verse 10:
➤ The Spirit descends upon Jesus in the form of a dove. The religious significance of doves is related to peace and reconciliation. The Spirit has to do with anointing, empowerment for action, and being equipped with the words of truth and revelation.

Verse11:
➤ The word from heaven is God's own self-affirmation of the identity of Jesus, and God's activity in and through him. It is not the case of what Jesus will be, but rather what he is. It is not the case that God will love him, but rather that God loves him; and it is not the case that God will be pleased with him, but rather that God is pleased with him.

We Apply the Word of God to Ourselves

WHAT CAN WE LEARN?
- As Jesus affirms John's ministry, we also need to acknowledge other people's gifts and ministries for mutual support.
- Jesus is God's emissary who does not discriminate against sinners, but rather identifies himself with them. And also came to save them.
- To be in Christ, with Christ, and for Christ, is to be a child of God. It is to be loved by God; it is to be a pleasure to God.
- All who are baptized in Christ are members of the same family and need not discriminate.
- It is Jesus who baptizes with the Holy Spirit. To be baptized by the Spirit of Jesus is to be immersed in his own life of love.

WHAT CAN WE CONFESS?
- We have discriminated against those we considered sinners, especially those infected by HIV/AIDS.
- We have put sin above the love of God in our relationship to God, in spite of the overwhelming abundance of biblical declarations to the contrary. It is love that deals with the reality of sin, and not sin demanding love as a ransom.
- We have often discriminated against women, who are also equal members of the body of Christ through baptism.

WHAT CAN WE BE THANKFUL FOR?
- For the example of Jesus;
- For the presence of the Holy Spirit to renew us;
- That when we repent, God is ready to forgive us for Christ's sake;
- That we can live a life that is considered sinless because past sins are covered by the blood of Jesus.

WHAT CAN WE PRAY FOR?
- For God's forgiveness for condemning and discriminating against people living with HIV/AIDS.

WHAT CAN WE FEEL?
- We feel accepted by Jesus who shows solidarity with sinners;
- We feel empowered by the Holy Spirit to live a life of loving solidarity.

WHAT CAN WE BE?
- God's children who are pleasing to him;
- People who are anointed and filled by the Holy Spirit.

WHAT CAN WE DO?
- We can bring assurance of God's love and forgiveness to those who are being discriminated against because they are HIV positive;
- We can educate ourselves and others about those who are infected with HIV;
- We can extend compassion to them and to the affected;
- We can provide care.

We Apply the Word to the Congregation/Society

The message from this passage is that God has forgiven sinners, and continues to forgive sinners as they come in repentance. Do members of the congregation accept those who are HIV positive, especially if they contracted the disease through promiscuity?

Song
Blessed Assurance, Jesus is mine.

Prayer

We are amazed, great God of glory, for the humility that Jesus Christ your Son, and our Lord and Savior demonstrated through his baptism. How he dared to identify himself with sinners, and by taking their sins upon himself broke the power of sin on humanity. As your people enter into his baptism, may they be liberated for all time from the power of sin upon their lives, families and communities. Forgive us when we have failed to identify with those in need of your cleansing among us. Help us to be agents of your grace. Through Jesus Christ our Lord. Amen

Suggested Objects/symbols/ideas: Water in a basin, a dove, carving of a fish, towel, white cloth.

By Augustine C. Musopule

3. Lord's Supper

SERVICE OF THE LORD'S SUPPER
Sermon Text: I Corinthians 11:23-24

Prayer

This is a service of communion and thanksgiving and we ask you to bless it. Due to the immense challenges we face in our lives, many of us are often tempted to think that there is little to be thankful for. We pray that this service will once again enable us to see the many blessings for which we can be thankful. We pray that through this service we will view our circumstances from a different light. The fact that some among us may be HIV positive is reason to be especially thankful for the gifts of life, fellowship and communion. Lord, we ask that as you issue an open invitation for us to sit at table with you, the church may work to undermine and combat all stigma against HIV positive people and other stigmatized groups in society. We pray that this service may inspire us to combat all practices - said and done -, which undermine community. In this service, we pray that we will be moved from chaos to community and fellowship with you, oh Lord, and with one another as human beings created in your image.

Song

Bind us together Lord,
Bind us together Lord,
Bind us with cords
That cannot be broken.

Bind us together Lord,
Bind us together Lord,
Bind us together with love.

There is only one Lord,
There is only one King.
(Anonymous, popular chorus)

Introduction

In many cultures - African cultures included - the sharing of a meal is the highest form of fellowship and communion. The sharing of a meal is the most basic and most central family ritual, in which members of the family engage. The invitation to a guest to share in the family meal is accordingly an important gesture of friendship and communion. It is significant that Jesus chose a meal as the best context for us to the remember him. As the time of his betrayal and crucifixion drew near, Jesus chose for farewell and remembrance purposes, the sharing of a meal. There is no better symbol of communion, friendship and fellowship than a meal. It is instructive that Jesus did not leave to chance the question of how he was to be remembered, but sought to give his disciples very concrete clues, guidelines and a very definite context. It is also instructive that Jesus chose a communal rather than an individual meal situation for the context of his remembrance. But we live in a world where meals - even family meal times - can no longer be taken for granted. In a world where some have more to eat than they can consume, there are millions who go for days without a decent meal. There are families for whom a decent family meal is a luxury that happens all too rarely. Effectively therefore, in the global meal table, there are millions who are excluded. What excludes them? Poverty; patriarchy; racism; sexism; HIV/AIDS. The stigmatization of HIV positive people. As long as the global meal table excludes some, the world is unable to witness to and remember Jesus Christ. We must be careful that the Holy Communion does not become just another of the many exclusive and immoral meals in which a few get nourished, when many are going hungry. Not only does Holy Communion remind us of a basic human act, but it also inspires us to work for a world in which there is genuine communion among all human beings, and between humans and God.

We Listen to the Word of God

We read I Corinthians 11:23-34

DETAILS OF THE TEXT
This passage is a recollection - it is Paul's recollection of the instructions from the Lord with regard to Holy Communion. For Paul, it is important that this practice be kept just as the Lord had commanded. Here, it is clearly the theological significance of the meal that is highlighted. The central theological message is that of linking the bread and the wine to the event of salvation. Human made bread and wine become (metaphors for) the broken body of the Christ and his shed blood. We must not pass too quickly over the fact and reality of the broken body and the spilt blood. These two theological truths find much resonance in the experience of many in Africa today. Diseases such as HIV/AIDS are breaking the body of Christ anew. Blood continues to be spilt in a world where the sanctity of life is no longer respected. The world is broken. So the theological significance and the subsequent theological controversies about Holy Communion should not blind us to its socio-economic and ethical significance of Holy Communion. Paul was very much awake to the latter. After reminding his readers of the words of the Lord, he proceeds to caution against unworthy eating of Holy Communion. He suggests introspection before Holy Communion and advises against gluttony or greed at the communion table. In our context of poverty and HIV/AIDS, we may have to revisit these words of caution, and conceptualize them and think anew of the things that make for communion and those that destroy it.

We Apply the Word of God

WHAT CAN WE LEARN?
- We learn that Jesus instructed that a simple communion meal is the context of his remembrance, and that he is best served and remembered in community.
- For communion to be real, all - including stigmatized and discriminated people - must be welcome unconditionally as God accepts us.
- Just as there are important theological issues in the practice and traditions surrounding Holy Communion, there are also ethical and socio-political issues.

WHAT DO WE HAVE TO CONFESS?
- We confess all the practices, policies and words that kill and stunt community.
- We confess the danger that Holy Communion can become one more meal of exclusion in a world where so many are excluded.
- We confess the exclusion of many - including HIV positive people - from the table of communion.
- We confess our silence in the face of massive stigmatization of HIV positive people, effectively cutting them off and denying them community and fellowship.

WHAT CAN WE BE THANKFUL FOR?
- We are thankful that, sinful as we are, we are made worthy to sit at table with the Lord.
- We are thankful that in a world full of divisions, discrimination and exclusion, we are all welcome to sit alongside one another and alongside Jesus Christ.
- We are thankful that Christ left us this ritual of community, fellowship and thanksgiving.

WHAT CAN WE PRAY FOR?
- We pray for an end to all that divides, discriminates and excludes.
- In a society where community is being torn apart by the HIV/AIDS pandemic, we pray for healing and for resilient community.
- We pray for a global table where no one is discriminated or excluded.
- We pray for a world where all have something to eat.

We Apply the Word of God to the Congregation

WHAT CAN WE FEEL?
- We feel ashamed at the extent of cruel and irrational stigma attached to HIV positive people.
- We feel compassionate towards all discriminated people.
- We feel anger at the abuse of Holy Communion, so it becomes one more meal of exclusion, rather than a context of community, witness and remembrance.
- We feel inspired by the realization that Jesus wants us to live in community with him.

WHAT CAN WE BE?
- We can be builders of community.
- We can be activists against discrimination and exclusion.

WHAT CAN WE DO?
- We can take action against stigmatization of HIV/AIDS sufferers.
- We can work towards making the communion table accessible to all within our own congregation.
- We can work for a global communion table that welcomes all and is able to supply nourishment to all.

Conclusion: A Word to Society

Holy Communion is a significant Christian ritual. In remembering the broken body of Christ, we recognize the broken world in which we live. We recognize the broken body of Christ - a body that is HIV positive. So we aught to pause to think of the things that break up our world and things that break up the church. We should think particularly of things that destroy and pervert genuine human community. In this ritual built around a most basic and community-inspiring human act, namely, the sharing of a meal, we are forced confess that in our world, even the sharing of a meal is fast becoming exclusive, as many go hungry. We are therefore challenged to name the policies and practices that break the world up and spill blood. We are challenged to work for a world in which there is real community. In such a world, stigma and discrimination will be eliminated. This is what it means to remember and to witness to Christ.

Prayer of Commitment
Lord, we thank you for allowing us to sit at the table with you. Give us strength to continue working for a world that is not broken - a world where blood is wantonly spilt. Help us to have courage to work for a world in which all have something to eat. Give us the vision and courage to build churches, which are home to strangers, the poor and the sick. We particularly ask you to make the church a home and refuge for HIV positive people. Above all we pray that you will enlist all of us in the fight against the spread of HIV/AIDS, poverty and discrimination.

Song
An appropriate song of community or Holy Communion may be sung.

Symbols/objects/ideas and commitments: The usual Holy Communion symbols will suffice.

By Tinyiko S. Maluleke

IAS FESTIVOS DA IGREJA

SANTA CEIA
Texto sugerido para o sermão: Lc 22:14-23

Oração

Obrigado Senhor por nos ter convidadona Tua Ceia. Sabemos que não somos dignos dela. Sabemos também que tu perdoas ao pecador que se arrepende. Por isso estamos aqui, para que nos fortaleças e purifiques. Cultive em nós o teu amor, para te servirmos com justiça, todos os dias da nossa vida.

Introdução

A Santa Ceia constituída por Jesus, é tomada pelos baptizados e confirmados. Nela, estão presentes o pão que simboliza o corpo de Cristo, e o vinho que simboliza o seu sangue. A igreja , corpo de Cristo, reúne-se à volta da mesa para tomar a Ceia até que Ele venha (I Co11.26). A doutrina de algumas igrejas proíbe a participação na Ceia a todos aqueles que tem problemas disciplinares. Os pecados cometidos por algumas pessoas não tem perdão pelo que, essas pessoas são interditas de tomá-la até à sua morte. Quando e como é que a igreja recebeu o poder para fazer isso? A ideia de que quem estiver contaminado (a) pelo HIV/SIDA é pecador (a), pressupõe que essas pessoas não podem também participar da S.Ceia. Será que pastores (as) padecendo desta doença não poderão mais tomá-la? Como entender esse comportamento quando a igreja fala de amor, perdão, justiça? O HIV/SIDA põe em causa a nossa pregação e convida-nos a uma reflexão profunda sobre as nossas atitudes porque, pelo baptismo, somos todos(as) um em Cristo (Gl 3.27).

Vamos Escutar a Palavra de Deus

Leia o texto. Sublinhe com um lápis as palavras mais importantes.

DETALHES
VV. 14-22
➢ Jesus toma a sua última Ceia com os seus discípulos. Nela anuncia a sua morte e a traição que será feita por um deles. Pede-lhes para ficarem a tomar a Ceia depois da sua partida, em sua memória.

V 23
➢ Os discípulos preocupados, tentam descobrir quem será o traidor.

QUE DEVEMOS CONFESSAR?
• Que nos púlpitos pregamos mentiras em vez do Evangelho da Boa Nova;
• Que muita gente afasta-se da igreja por culpa nossa;
• Que discriminamos aqueles a quem Deus mais quer no seu Reino.

CANÇÂO
Escolher uma que esteja de acordo com o tema

ORAÇÂO

Senhor omnipotente, agradecemos-te pelo imenso amor que tens por nós. Quiseste que participássemos da tua glória. Convidaste-nos e continuas a convidar-nos no teu banquete, porque queres dividir tudo connosco. Quem somos nós para merecer tamanha consideração? Senhor, o teu amor e justiça, tornam-nos indignos de sermos chamados teus filhos. Tu não nos sentencias à morte, mas nós somos implacáveis para condenar os (as) outros (as). O que é pior, é que colocamos barreiras intransponíveis para aqueles (as) que querem aproximar-se de ti. Perdoa-nos Senhor. Transforme os nossos empedernidos corações, e faça deles vasos de bênção, que levam Boas Novas aos que delas necessitam, em nome do Teu Filho Jesus Cristo. Amen

Objectos: Desenho ou fotografia de alguém a oferecer pão a outrém.

Por: Felicidade N. Cherinda

4. Good Friday and Easter

GOOD FRIDAY
Sermon Text: Mark 15:16-41

Introduction

Many people in Sub-Saharan Africa live with untold sufferings. At the moment there is famine of a magnitude that has not been experienced in a long while in Southern Africa. Children and adults are dying of starvation. Others have had to resort to practices like immigration and sex work in order to make ends meet. Parents have to watch helplessly as their children die from malnutrition and related diseases. Many of these are Christians, and they have been told that if they are faithful and pray hard enough things will be okay. But things have not been, despite their fidelity to the Christian faith. Consequently they ask, *"Where is God when it hurts most?"*

We Listen to the Word of God

DETAILS OF THE TEXT
Mark's narrative of Jesus' arrest, trial, crucifixion and death is made up of numerous individual scenes, each of which is appropriate for a Good Friday Sermon. It might be advisable for the preacher to isolate and focus on one particular aspect of the narrative. The narrative is full of irony. The soldiers tease and mock Jesus with the words, 'Long live king of the Jews!' They even create a crown of thorns for him. Little did they know that in fact, this was the King of Kings and the Lord of the Lords! The divine plan was taking effect in the foolish act of human beings poking and mocking God. Here God, in the person of Jesus, took on the form of a servant and was beaten so that we may be saved. God took upon human suffering.

67

We Apply the Word of God to Ourselves

Christians worship a crucified God who is not removed from their experiences. God experiences the shame and the pain of HIV/AIDS.

WHAT CAN WE LEARN?
Christ's body, which was spat on, whipped and broken for us, takes shape in the emaciated bodies of Africa children who die from AIDS everyday. God is there when it hurts most, not in heaven, but in our suffering.

We need to ask ourselves about the image of God that we portray in our theologies and in our pulpits. Is it a God who is far removed from people's experiences, a grandfather up in the sky, or is it a God whose body we see broken in the bodies of sex workers, who are abused every night, in children who are orphaned daily, and women who infected through rape?

WHAT CAN WE CONFESS?
- We have not always been empathetic to the poor and down trodden;
- We have portrayed an image of God that is triumphal even through the Bible testifies to God whose body was broken for us;
- We have stigmatized those who have HIV/AIDS, failing to see God in their faces.

WHAT CAN WE BE THANKFUL FOR?
- Jesus Christ and what he did for us on the cross;
- Theologians who challenge us to re-visit our images of God so that they can be true to the New Testament;
- The opportunity to celebrate Good Friday.

Prayer

Leader: Crucified God we come to you with bruised memories and sorrows.

Response: Listen to our prayers for we pray in the name of Jesus Christ.

Leader: God who was ridiculed, spat on, and whose body starves with no access to food.

Response: We bring your orphaned children to our communities. They live without their mothers and fathers, but we know you look after them.

Leader: We bring before you the pain of those who starve and have no access to food.

Response: We trust you to provide us with our daily bread, as you did to our parents and their parents before them. Bring us rain and turn our dusty fields into bountiful blessings of food.

Leader: Christ our liberator rescues us from the forces of death, which surrounds us; such as rape, domestic violence, sex industry and HIV/AIDS.

Response: Oh Lord, restore us to yourself we pray. Raise among us men and women who will together resist these forces for your name's sake.

All: Crucified God be part of our sorrows.
Weep with us and wipe away our tears.
May our brokenness find healing in you,
And may we take delight in your cross.
Amen

Song

When I survey the wondrous cross,
On which the Prince of Glory died,
My richest gain I count but loss,
And pour contempt on all pride.

Forbid it, Lord, that I should boast,
Save in the death of Christ my God,
All the vain things that charm me most,
I sacrifice them to his blood.

See from his head, his hands, and his feet,
Sorrow and love flow mingled down,
Did e'er such a sorrow meet,
Or thorns compose of rich a crown?

His dying crimson, like a robe,
Spreads o'er his body on the tree;
Then I am dead to all the globe is dead to me.

Was the whole realm of nature mine?
That was a present far too small;
Love so amazing, so divine,
Demands my soul, my life, and my all.
(© Isaac Watts)

Suggested Object/symbols/ideas: The worshiper could use a big cross and place it in the central place, so that it becomes a focal point. Next to it could be a little candle.

By Moiseraele P. Dibeela

5. Resurrection/Restoration

RESURRECTION
Sermon Text: Luke 24: 1

Introduction

Whether death (as a tragedy) has come out of preventable, postponable or manageable conditions or whether (as a miracle) it has come out of our natural end (Genesis 23:1-2, 25: 7-8, 35:28-29), the resurrection truth reminds us that our God transforms our death into eternal life, if we believe in God's son, Jesus (John 11:25-26) and if we are faithful to him in love and repentance. In the context of HIV/AIDS, the resurrection story has three-fold significance:

- We should never tire from preventing and postponing all preventable and postponeable suffering and death. But once we reach the end of the road; we should embrace inevitable sufferings and death with a sense of hope and victory (I Corinthians 15:3-58; I Thessalonians 4:4-13);

- What may look impossible with our human eyes, minds and hearts is possible with God (Luke 24: 2,5,6);

- We should never allow preventable, postponable and manageable deaths to happen simply because we want ourselves or our loved ones to have eternal life quickly. It is quite inappropriate to use the resurrection story as a death recipe or prescription – as if it is always good to allow, invent or increase trouble to maximize good!

We Listen to the Word of God

Read or choose someone to read the Luke 24:1;
Read the three other reports about Christ's resurrection on Sunday morning
(Mark 16:1-8, Matthew 28:1-10, John 20:1-9);
Explain that the reports supplement each other.

DETAILS OF THE TEXT
Verse 1:
➢ "Now upon the first day of the week, very early in the morning, they came into the sculpture, bringing spices, which they had prepared…."
Have you ever been scolded or reprimanded for doing something which humanly speaking looks like a waste of effort, energy, time and resources? For example they say,
 -"Do not bother, he will soon be dead anyway,"
 -"Do not waste your money and your time, that patient, child, family, community, nation, or continent is beyond resuscitation/recovery/rehabilitation!"

Verse 55:
➢ It tells us that the women followed the men that were carrying the body of Jesus; that they saw the men put Jesus in a tomb and roll a very big stone on the entrance. They probably

also saw the soldiers being deployed on the site to ensure nobody tampered with the burial of Jesus. Nevertheless, they went ahead (according to v. 56) to prepare spices and ointments and after the Sabbath, took them early Sunday morning to the tomb, supposedly to anoint the body. What a faith!

Verse 2:
➤ "And they found the stone rolled away…"! (Miracle 1)

Verse 3:
➤ "And they entered in and found not the body of the Lord Jesus. (Miracle 2)

Verse 5:
➤ "Why are you seeking the living among the dead? (Note that important question)

Verse 6:
➤ "He is not here, but he is risen." (attestation of a miracle)

We Apply the Word of God to Ourselves

WHAT CAN WE LEARN
- The women's faith is amazing!
- Jesus' resurrection story gives us hope to face and confront a hopeless situation.
- We have hope to live beyond the grave, because of Jesus own resurrection.

WHAT DO WE HAVE TO CONFESS?
- We are often paralyzed by seemingly hopeless situations and are easily discouraged/distracted from action in faith. We confess faithlessness and hopelessness in face of trails and problems.

WHAT CAN WE BE THANKFUL FOR?
- For the resurrection of Jesus, the writing of the story, and the faith and courage displayed by the women. All are an inspiration to our own faith, hope and struggles.
- That we can also resurrect from our fear and hopelessness.

WHAT CAN WE PRAY FOR?
- That the resurrection story may be preached powerfully and joyfully in the whole world.
- That those doing something about HIV/AIDS be encouraged, for, "What may seem impossible in the eyes, minds and hearts of people, is possible with God."

We Apply the Word of God to the Congregation, Society and the World

WE LOOK AT THE SITUATION OF OUR LISTENERS.
- As people face the struggles of living with HIV/AIDS, does the church reflect the hope, faith and assurance generated by the resurrection story?

- God implores us not to kill, whether that killing is by a bullet, a spear, or by behaviors and actions that lead to the spread HIV/AIDS. Yet the same God does not become powerless over our ungodly acts of murder or suicide. God sets right what has fallen. God shows us what has been messed up, and resurrects what has been denied from life, through our individual and collective acts of omission and commission.

WE PREACH THE GOSPEL

- In spite of HIV/AIDS, the living God of the miracle of resurrection still exists. God suffers with us (Hebrews 2:9). We are not alone with struggle against HIV/AIDS (II Corinthians 1:1-18). God promises to be present with us in our struggle (Philemon 3:10) and promises us victory over temporal suffering now and in eternity (Romans 8:18, 21:1-5).

- The resurrection is God's seal that Jesus really died for us, that he really lives, and that one-day he will raise the dead and take the believers (whether they died of AIDS or any other condition) to heaven.

Song

He is Lord, (2x)
He is risen from the dead, and he is Lord,
Every knee shall bow, every tongue confess
That Jesus Christ is Lord.
He is peace;
He is life;
He is love;
He is health;
He is God;
He is Joy.
(Anonymous)

Prayer
To be recited by all

Dear Lord, your resurrection gives us hope, courage and trust knowing that you transformed death into life. When the road of life is hard, when it leads to the grave, let us rest in the assurance that beyond the grave, you will be waiting for us in your glory. Lord helps us to travel life's road faithfully in the comfort and hope of resurrection.
AMEN!

Suggested Objects: Candles, Stones, pebbles.

By Canon Gideon Byamugisha

RESURRECTION
Sermon Text: Mark 16:1-8

Introduction

The resurrection is central to Christianity. A comparative analysis of the world's religious traditions shows that the theme of Christ's resurrection is crucial to Christianity's self-understanding. This theme is valuable in HIV/AIDS prevention and care. Christ's victory over death implies that the high death rate due to HIV/AIDS is contrary to God's promise of abundant life.

In our African setting where HIV/AIDS has almost resulted in a culture of death, the resurrection becomes a useful symbol. It should send out a message of hope to millions of disillusioned communities. As communities stagger under weight of pain and death, the resurrection should awaken flagging spirits. The good news that life triumphs over death should resurrect dead convictions. Thus, the story of the resurrection should reinvigorate communities to act decisively against HIV/AIDS. We must resurrect against the invasion of death in our families, villages, nations and continent.

We Listen to the Word of God

The women in the story possessed immense faith and love. At this point, you can introduce the local requirements associated with post-burial rituals. The women in the story also recognized the enormity of the task before them and deliberated amongst themselves, formulating viable strategies. You should also highlight the fact that after the discovery of the resurrection, a sense of mission followed. In the context of HIV/AIDS, concrete planning and specific responses are called for.

We Apply the Word of God to Ourselves

WHAT CAN WE BE THANKFUL FOR?
- Some leaders and individuals have actively participated in programmes to fight HIV/AIDS, and have resurrected communal hope.
- That many people carry the message of hope to their sick and bed-laden patients.

WHAT CAN WE LEARN?
- Like the women who were not discouraged, we need to play our part in HIV/AIDS prevention and care.
- It is possible for us to be afraid of the challenge.
- HIV/AIDS should stir us into action.

WHAT DO WE HAVE TO CONFESS?
- Failure to preach a message of life and hope.
- That sometimes we are paralyzed by the HIV/AIDS challenge.
- That death does not have the final say.

We Apply the Word of God to the Congregation

- Highlight the fact that resurrection should also be applied to communities ravaged by HIV/AIDS.
- Draw attention to the fact that the women brainstormed on their way to the tomb. Congregations need to plan in order to be effective in fighting HIV/AIDS.
- The symbol of resurrection communicates God's choice of life over death.

Conclusion: A Word on Society

Resurrection stories indicate the possibility of communities being totally transformed. The paralysis induced by the epidemic should be countered by a theology of hope. This is based on the conviction that in raising Christ from the dead, God was affirming life. Society is therefore called upon to combat all systems that stifle life and promote death. This includes fighting poverty, gender inequalities, corrupt governments, abuse of children, international injustice and oppressive cultures.

Song

He is Lord, (x2)

He has risen from the dead and he is Lord.

(CLG Hymn Book, No. 54)

Or

Akamuka vakangoona machira chete (x2)
Kwakangosara machira chete
(© Charles Charamba)

Prayer

All praise and honor be yours,
Lord of wondrous works.
While we were yet sinners,
You sacrificed your only begotten son
Jesus Christ, to atone for our arrogance and disobedience.
By your might, you raised him from the dead.
You delivered him from the jaws of death,
That we may have life, and have it abundantly.
Because Jesus lives, we can face tomorrow.
We are comforted and empowered.
May the Holy Spirit minister to us.
May the empty tomb generate confidence in us,
To recognize that life triumphs over death.
Strengthen us to walk in your holy path,
To the glory of your name. Amen

Poem

"HE HAS RISEN, HE IS NOT HERE" (Mark 16:6)

A rolled back stone;

An empty tomb;

This is my story;

This is my song.

In his absence I became;

In his new being I rejoice;

I too will go and tell

The tale of our salvation,

This foolishness avails life;

This scandal heals hurts;

This mystery explains;

God's salvation history.

Broken are the chains of slavery;

Chained are the jaws of death;

Charged is the hope for life eternal;

For he is risen, and he lies not where they placed him!

He has defeated HIV/AIDS;

He has ignited communal hope;

Life has overcome death.

© Ezra Chitando

Prayer

The Lord's Prayer, *by all.*

Suggested objects/symbols/ideas: Torn garments (resurrection); a painting of empty tomb, any thriving indigenous plant.

By Ezra Chitando

6. Ascension

Sermon Text: Luke 24:50-53

Call to worship

Leader: "When the Spirit of truth comes, that Spirit will guide you into all the truth; for the Spirit will not speak independently, but will speak whatever the Spirit hears and will declare to you the things that are to come. The Spirit will glorify me by taking what is mine and declaring it to you" (John 16:11-15).

All: Fill us with your Spirit of power, the Spirit that enables us to speak. Enkindle us with your Spirit, the Spirit of fire and power.

Opening Song

Munezero munezero
(Thuma Mina, No. 17)

Scripture Reading: Luke 24:50-53

"Then Jesus led them out as far as Bethany, and with uplifted hands, Jesus blessed them. While blessing them, Jesus withdrew from them and was carried up into heaven. And they worshiped Jesus, and returned to Jerusalem with great joy and they were continually in the temple blessing God."

Time for Interpretation and Songs

Instructions: If you are holding a Bible study for a small group such as: Sunday school class, youth group or mothers union, get your participants to sit in a circle. Have each one person read the text and then let each person have the opportunity to interpret the meaning of the passage in relation to the HIV/AIDS epidemic and various other social evils that confront us. If it is in the general service, read the passage and open the interpretation to anyone who wishes to speak. The rest of the listeners can participate in the interpretation by interjecting with a relevant song between the different interpreters. If the participants wish, they can dance to these songs. This liturgy is communal and openly participatory, allowing all the members who wish, the right to interpret the word. It is also a pure celebration in praise of God with multiple songs and dance. Lastly, this loosely organized liturgy attempts to capture the worship style of many African Christian churches: their liturgy is communal, a joyous celebration in song, dance and drum, and it is oral— not written.

Sharing the Water of Life

"Those who drink of the water that I will give them, will never be thirsty. The water that I will give, will become in them a spring of water gushing up to eternal life."

Participants are invited to share the water of life.

Closing Song

Sizohamba naye
(Thuma Mina, No. 180)

Closing Prayer

Loving and caring God, we thank you for the fellowship of the Holy Spirit that fills us with joy. It fills us with power, the power that heals our bodies and soul. We thank you for your peace, for it surpasses all understanding. You give us peace in the midst of all that troubles. We thank you for your ascension, your rising above the power of death. We know that no death of body, mind and spirit can keep us down. We live in joy because you rose from death. Help us to dwell in the joy and fire of your Spirit at all times. Help us to ascend through your resurrection power. This we pray, in Jesus name. Amen

By Musa W. Dube

7. World AIDS Day

Sermon Text: Isaiah 65:17-23

Introduction

With millions of people already dead, and millions of others either living with, or personally affected by HIV/AIDS; the epidemic constitutes one of the most critical problems for our time. Religious institutions in general, and churches in particular, have very important roles to play in fighting the spread of the disease from one person to the other; in mobilizing care and treatment for those already infected and in mitigating the effects of the disease on the families, communities and the nations that have been affected.

World AIDS Day is a special event for churches. By celebrating this day through worship, prayers, praise, word and testimony; individual Christians and whole congregations are helped to:

- Consolidate the "caring church" concept within their activities and plans.

- Break down barriers of prejudice, fear, stigma, and complacency which still hinder our open discussion about and practical action against the disease - AIDS.

- Acquire more spiritual and social strength, and resources to fight the disease and its determinant factors.

- The practice of listening to God's word and the discipline of prayer have always been very important dimensions of our spirituality, but they are even more imperative today given the increased burden of diseases, poverty, famine and conflicts in our families, communities and amongst our nations. World AIDS Day gives us both the opportunity and responsibility to ask for, and find God's mercy, grace and help in this critical time of need.

Isaiah 65: 17-23

We Listen to the Word of God

Read or choose someone to read the Isaiah 65:17-23.

DETAILS OF THE TEXT
The Israelites were living in hurting conditions. Diseases, suffering and early death was the order of the day, for both those who were in exile and those who had escaped complicity. God wanted to bring this to a stop.

Verse 17:
➢ "For behold, I create new heavens and a new earth; and the former shall not be remembered nor come to mind." Note the phrase "I create," which is a present continuous. He is not saying, "I will create," but rather "I create," today and tomorrow, this and next week, this and the next year.

Verse 19:
➢ "And the voice of weeping shall no more be heard, nor the voice of crying."
The pain, suffering and death caused by HIV/AIDS and other social evils tare the heart of God, and moved God to action. God is concerned about the declining life spans. Maternal and paternal morbidity and mortality rates from preventable and manageable conditions are a concern to God.

Verses 20-23:
➢ Describes the new creation and the living environment, as God wills it to be.

We Apply the Word of God to Ourselves

WHAT CAN WE LEARN?
- God has already decided, HIV/AIDS must go! All the prophecies of the Old Testament, and all the sayings of Jesus, testify to a God who loves life and is grieved by anything that reduces the quality of life. World AIDS Day, in its self is an occasion to learn what God says about our duty to fight the HIV/AIDS epidemic.
- We need to work with God to eliminate HIV/AIDS.

WHAT DO YOU CONFESS?
- In our roles and responsibilities as individuals, fathers, mothers, millers, educators, political leaders, spiritual advisors, youth leaders, peers, technical resources persons, service providers, planners, etc, we have not thought of or done all that we are supposed to do in order to bring about good health as God intended it to be at individual, family, local community, national, regional and global level.

WHAT CAN WE BE THANKFUL FOR?
- God wills that we live long, productive and fruitful lives even when reality seems to suggest the contrary;
- We still have a chance to make a difference.

WHAT CAN WE PRAY FOR?
- That God's will for our individual and collective lives come to pass through improved physical, economic, social practical and spiritual ordering of our lives at all levels – individual, family, local community, national, regional and global.
- That we become instruments to God's will.
- That God gives us the serenity to accept things and situations we may not be able to change, both in our lives and these of our loved ones.

We Apply the Word of God to the Congregation, Society and the World

WE LOOK AT THE SITUATION OF OUR LISTENERS
Verse 19:
➢ Many are weeping and crying.

Verse 20:
➢ Many are dying at very young ages.

Verse 21:
➢ Many are building houses and homes, but die before inhabiting them.

Verse 22:
➢ Many are not reaping the fruits of their labour.

Verse 23:
➢ Many are bringing forth children for trouble (orphans, child headed households, rape, defilement, lack of education opportunities, world/ regional religious/tribal conflicts, hunger, moral degeneration, lack of love for neighbour and God, etc).

WE PREACH GOD'S LAW
- We need to cooperate with God (we are co–creators), in bringing about this kingdom on earth through individual and societal reflection, repentance and rededication to a just, fair and healthier world order.

WE PREACH THE GOSPEL
- Jesus backed Isaiah's prophecy by declaring that, "He came that we may have life in its fullness." This is good news (gospel), although it is not yet good news for the majority of population which is collapsing under the burden of preventable and manageable illness, and other negative socio-economic/political conditions.

- We need to develop goals, strategies and action plans as individuals, and as church groups to help change these negative conditions, prevent new HIV infections, look after the sick, advocate for increased and fairer treatment services, and mitigate the impact of the diseases on the families, institutions, local communities and nations.

Since God is always on the side of life (Romans 8), God will surely support all our efforts in this endeavor.

Song
"United Against AIDS"

Chorus: United against AIDS,;

Unite and be safe,
Get the facts and get to know what AIDS is all about.

We want to thank all those that give in their lives,
They stand firm to fight AIDS and
Not people with AIDS.

Chorus: United against AIDS;

So many brothers and sisters,
Relatives and friends,
Have left us and many are to go,
We must stop the trend.

Chorus: United against AIDS;

So many friends reject us,
But why neglect us,
Why do you go away, why do you leave us,
When we are so close?

Chorus: United against AIDS;

So many times we are worried,
And sometimes we are crying,
Lets stand together to fight,
Until we reach the end!

Chorus: United against AIDS;

So let us all get together,
And encourage us,
Together we stand and fight until we reach the end. (3x)

(Hasifa Nanfuka, Taso Masaka. Reproduced with permission from, The caring: World AIDS Campaign: Special Prayer Service Liturgy, "Diocese of Namirembe.")

Prayer

Lord God, during this World AIDS Day:
We repent of our denial, complacency and failure towards the HIV/AIDS epidemic.
We are re-committing ourselves to communicating God's grace to the world;
To ministering, responding to, and identifying with those in need.

We give up our feelings of self–righteousness, our judgmental attitudes and our faulty beliefs about the HIV/AIDS diseases and the people living with it. Open our hearts for change and for forgiveness. Provide power to those who will bring change at the individual, family, institutional, local community, national and global level.

Enable us to promote positive examples of righteous, safe and healthy living in our cultural, social, sexual, reproductive, political and spiritual lives. Strengthen our families, communities, and nations by removing neglect, conflict and individualism. As we light this candle as a sign of our re-dedication to HIV/AIDS work; help us to listen, to learn and to live. In Jesus' name we pray. Amen

A Candle is lit.

Suggested Objects /symbols/ideas: Candles, badges and t-shirts bearing reminders, Bibles, photographs/posters and leaflets. People living with HIV/AIDS can also give their testimonies.

By Canon Gideon Byamugisha

Part 3
Themes for General Services

1. Life
      Genesis 1-2 (Musa W. Dube)
      Genesis 1-2 (Ezra Chitando)
      Mark 1:40-45 (Felicidade N. Cherinda)

2. Compassion
      Matthew 25:31-46 (Musa W. Dube)
      Luke 13:10-17 (Canon Gideon Byamugisha) (Felicidade N. Cherinda)

3. Hope
      Ezekiel 37:1-13 (Tinyiko S. Maluleke)
      Ezra 1:1-11 (Ezra Chitando)
      Mark 5:21-43 (Isabel Apawo Phiri)

4. Repentance
      Luke 18:9-14 (Moiseraele P. Dibeela)

5. Forgiveness
      Luke 7:36-50 (Augustine C. Musopule)

6. Love
      I Corinthians 13:1-13 (Augustine C. Musopule)

7. Fear and Desperation
      II Kings 6:24-30 (Isabel Apawo Phiri)

8. Stigma and Discrimination
      Job 3:1-26 (Augustine C. Musopule)
      John 9:1-4 (Moiseraele P. Dibeela)
      Leviticus 12:1-8 and 15: 19-24 (Faluta L. Moyo)

9. Sexuality
      Songs of Songs 1:1-7 (Tinyiko S. Maluleke)
      Songs of Songs 7:1-13 (Ezra Chitando)
      Songs of Songs 8:1-10 (Canon Gideon Byamugisha)

10. Reconciliation
      Luke 15:11-32 (Tinyiko S. Maluleke)

11. Healing
      Mark 1:40-42 and Luke: 7:20-22 (Musa W. Dube)

1. Life

LIFE: "IN THE BEGINNING…"
Sermon Text: Genesis 1-2

Instructions: If you are in an average to small sized study group (Sunday school, women's, men's and youth meetings) use one Bible to read Genesis 1-2. Let each person read two verses and pass it on, until the story is finished. Then ask each person to comment about what they think of the verses they read. If you are preaching in a larger and more formal service, arrange for dancers, ululation, those who will whistle and drummers. For scripture reading, get different readers to read the creation story either as compiled below, or from their Bibles. They should read their verses where they are seated. The idea is that the creation story must be experienced, and the creating word of God should come alive in recreating the worshippers. For the worship area, you can choose symbols and objects that portray the diversity of life in God's creation; such as cloth of many colors, plants, water, flowers, etc—whatever is useful, available and acceptable in your context and faith background.

Opening Dance

A dance of vitality in praise to God, and celebration of God's gift of the life that each one of us embodies. This dance can/should be in the local dance styles—as God gave your particular people to express their joy in a dance form.

Call to Worship

Leader:	You are the well of living waters;
All:	Quench our thirst with your waters of life.
Leader:	You are the bread of life;
All:	Feed us and fill our hunger for life.
Leader:	You are the resurrection and life;
All:	Raise us from the valley of dry bones, breathe life into our hopeless bodies.

Song

Oh Lord My God, when I am in awesome wonder
Or any appropriate song on creation and life.

Introduction

If there is one thing that HIV/AIDS surely attacks, it is human life. With 40 million people currently infected, 22 million dead, 13 million children orphaned, and many more getting infected daily, it is undoubted that HIV/AIDS trivializes life. Beyond physical death, HIV/AIDS has also undertaken a severe attack on spiritual, psychological and economic life. Some may have suffered and died physically, but worst is that the majority—families, communities and countries, died internally and mentally when they lost hope for the future. The quality of life has been severely reduced for both the infected and the affected.

It is therefore important to revisit how and why life was created, and what it was meant to be. We note that in Genesis 1-2, all life was created by God, and it was created good. We need to reclaim our right to life from the plunder of HIV/AIDS. We need to reclaim our right to live a good life. We need to heal and resurrect our communities from fear, hopelessness and HIV/AIDS stigma. We need to also address those social evils that fuel HIV/AIDS; such as poverty and gender inequalities, by assessing how the creation story addresses these issues. What are God's values on social justice? Since God created life, the HIV/AIDS attack on life violates the will of God. Further, since God gave human beings access to resources (Genesis 1:29), poverty which is the number one sponsor of HIV/AIDS, violates God's will.

We Listen to the Word of God

A participatory and poetic reading: Genesis 1-2

Reader 1:
In the beginning when God created the heavens and the earth,
The earth was formless and void...
Then God said, "Let there be light."
And there was light…

ALL*:* And God saw that the light was good;

Reader 2:
And God said, "Let there be a dome in the midst of waters…"
"Let the waters under the sky be gathered together in one place,
And let the dry land appear".
And it was so.

ALL: And God saw that it was good;

Reader 3:
Then God said, "Let the earth put forth vegetation,
Plants yielding seed and fruit trees of every kind on earth,"
And it was so.

ALL: And God saw that it was good;

Reader 4:
And God said, "Let there be lights in the dome of the sky…
Let them be for signs and for seasons and for days and years…"
And it was so…

ALL: And God saw that it was good;

Reader 5:
And God said, "Let the waters bring forth swarms of living creatures,

Let the birds fly above the earth across the dome of the sky…"
So God created….

ALL:
And God saw that it was good,
And God said, "Let the earth bring forth living creatures of every kind…"
And it was so.

ALL: And God saw that it was good;

Reader 6:
Then God said, "Let us make humankind
In our image, according to our likeness…"
So God created humankind in God's own image,
In the image of God, God created them,
Male and female God created them…

ALL: God blessed them…

Reader 7:
And God said, be fruitful and multiply,
And fill the earth and subdue it,
And have dominion over the fish of the sea,
And over the birds of the air,
And over every living thing that moves upon the earth,
God said, 'See, I have given you,
Every plant yielding seed that is upon the face of the earth,
And every tree with see in its fruit,
You shall have them for food…
And it was so.

ALL:
God saw everything that God had made,
And indeed it was VERY good.
In celebration and praise of the creator God of life:

Ululation: All women or selected individuals
Whistling: All men or selected men
Drumming: Play the drum/s

DETAILS OF THE TEXT
Verses 1-2:
  ➢ God is depicted as creator of both heavens and the earth. God can be seen as builder, artist or mother, who brings life to life.

  ➢ Note that the earth was formless and covered by darkness, and God brings order to it.

Verses 3-13:

➢ "Then God said, 'Let there be light'" and there was light. Up to verse 5, and for the whole first day of creation, God focused on creating light. Two points are notable here.

➢ First, the first act of bringing shape to the earth is the creation of light. Why light? We associate light with vision and God's salvation. It enables comprehension and nurtures life. Light embodies a spark of God's creative power and vision upon all life.

➢ Second, God creates through God's word. The word is powerful, so powerful its very utterance is realized in a concrete event or object, as this is confirmed by the phrase 'and it was so.' How can we let God's creative and powerful word continue to light the earth and to recreate the formlessness and darkness that hovers over our earth and souls?

➢ In verse 6-9 the creation of things (sky, seas, dry land) by word continues, bringing order into the earth. Note that it ends with an evaluation, "And God saw that it was good." As a creator, artist, builder and mother, God is very interested in the end product. God evaluates it and appreciates it until God is satisfied with its quality, "God saw that it was good!" Highlight that God insists that we must not only have life, but also have it in fullness. (John 10:10)

In verses 11-13, the creation of living things begins. God creates plant life, and again, "God saw that it was good." The latter must be underlined.

Verses 14-25:

➢ Creation of stars, seasons, years, moon and the sun. Note, once more, this is through the power of God's word, "Let there be... and it was so." Note again, that this is also closed by an evaluation, "And God saw that it was good," (v.18). Every part of the creation was created with much care, love and artistic vigor. God did not proceed to another stage before God was sure that what was done was done well—it was good!

➢ In verses 20-23 God begins to create animal life and this closes with the same evaluation, "And God saw that it was good." This repetition is emphatic on God's intention, care, love and artistic vigor that accompanied the whole creation. Nothing was of less value. The quality of life is a must for the whole creation.

➢ Note that animals are blessed and given the right to multiply.

Verses 26-27:

➢ Note that God begins to create human life—as the very last form of life to be created. God says, "Let us make humankind in our image." Three points are notable here:

➢ First, note the communal invitation phrase "let us make" as opposed to "let there be" which has accompanied the creation of other forms of life. Why this change? Who are the subjects addressed by God? The heavens are populated by angels or the heavenly council (Job 38:7; I Kings 22:19; Jeremiah 23:18-23) and to the Christians, God is the Triune God. The creation of human being is a communal and consultative.

➤ Second, the phrase, 'in our image' is notable. While the Bible discourages any physical representation of God, human beings are said to be created to in God's image, in God's 'likeness.' What does this mean? What are the implications? How are we created in God's image?

➤ Emphasize that the whole humankind, all people, were created in God's image and likeness, regardless of their race, ethnicity, gender, ability/disability, culture, class, age, sexual orientation, etc. Discrimination on the basis of any form of human difference or identity violates the Creator God, who saw it fit that all people should be created in God's own image and likeness. This verse allows us to support the human rights of all and to fight all forms of oppression.

➤ Verse 27 in particular, singles out that biological sex, men and women, were both created in God's image and likeness. Given that gender, a cultural construction, has been used to authorize the discrimination of women—this verse need to be underlined. In particular, given that gender inequalities are a major driving force behind the spread of HIV/AIDS, it is important to underline that men and women were created equal and that our families, churches and communities must embrace the empowerment of both sexes.

Verses 28-29:

➤ Verse 28 is notable. Human beings are blessed and given the power to multiply and fill the earth. This is the mandate to reproduce. It authorizes the right to live and have children. In the HIV/AIDS context, this blessings needs to be recaptured. However, it must not be used to promote unsafe sex, or to discourage abstinence, where married women are forced to have children with HIV positive men. The quality of life remains important in multiplication.

➤ "Fill the earth and subdue it and have dominion over it," is notable. Due to their being made in God's image, human beings are given a unique responsibility in "God's created world." They are custodians and stewards of God's earth, charged with the role of keeping the earth good. This leadership position and role in the earth community. Both men and women, all people of all races, and ethnic groups are given this role.

➤ This latter point needs to be underlined, for HIV/AIDS particularly, those groups who are denied leadership and decision-making roles, such as women, despised ethnic groups and races, disabled/physically challenged people, people of different sexual orientation, children and people living with HIV/AIDS (PLWHAs). Underline that it is God's will for all people to have both leadership and decision power in God's world and order.

➤ In verse 29, "God said, see I have given you every plant... for food." Access to God's resources is extended to all. *No one should be poor.* Underline that poverty is a violation of God's will for all people. Why are some people poor? Who and what hinders their God given right to have access to God's resources? Whatever answer that we give, let us fight poverty for it is not God's will for anyone.

➤ Highlight that in the HIV/AIDS era, it is poverty that ranks as the number one sponsor of the epidemic. It hinders both prevention and provision of quality care. The church must, therefore, fight and condemn poverty.

Verses 30-31:
- ➤ God cares for animals too and provides for them. Animals have rights to the resources of the earth. God has given them, "every green plant for food."

- ➤ Highlight that God's creation ends with a final and emphatic overall evaluation, "God saw everything that God had made, and indeed, it was *very* good". (v. 31)

- ➤ Underline that the latter calls us all, the members of the earth community, to keep God's creation balanced, good, interdependent and blessed, according to the blessings that were given to all members of the earth community. The right that we all have is the right to life - quality life. Life must be good, for God meant it to be *very good!*

We Apply the Word of God to Ourselves

WHAT CAN WE LEARN?
- That all life is sacred;
- That all things were created good, in diversity and interconnected;
- That both men and women were created in God's image, both were blessed, both were given leadership roles and access to the resources of the earth;
- Animal and environmental rights have a place in our Christian theology.

WHAT DO WE HAVE TO CONFESS?
- That we have not kept the earth, the whole creation good;
- We have not always seen diversity as God's creative hand;
- We have not always seen and worshipped God through creation;
- We have not always affirmed that all people were created in God's image;
- Many people are denied leadership and decision making roles;
- Many millions have no access to the resources of the earth, they live in poverty.

WHAT CAN WE BE THANFUL FOR?
- That God created all life good and all human beings in God's image;
- That all human beings were given leadership and access to resources.

WHAT CAN WE PRAY FOR?
To remember that:
- Our role as God's custodians is to keep the earth and everything good;
- No person should be poor, for God gave the earth resources to all;
- No one should be denied leadership and decision making power, for God gave all of us custodianship over the earth resources, including HIV/AIDS drugs;
- No person should be denied their human rights in life, since God created all of us in God's own image and likeness.

We Apply the Word of God to the Congregation

WHAT CAN WE FEEL?
- That life is beautiful and artistic and must be celebrated and enjoyed;
- Repentant for failing to maintain the goodness of creation and for not being champions of women's, environmental and animal rights.

WHAT CAN WE BE?
- Custodians and stewards of God's creation;
- Speakers of the creative and powerful Word of God.

WHAT CAN WE DO?
- Work with relevant NGOs for the protection of environment, to protect human rights, to reduce poverty, to protect women's rights and all the oppressed groups.
- Undertake various projects that fight HIV/AIDS' attack on life.

Conclusion: A Word on Society

HIV/AIDS is an epidemic within other social epidemics of poverty; gender inequalities; national corruption; discrimination on the basis of race, ethnicity, age, sexuality, ability/disability; and international injustice that promotes economic depravation and hinders access to HIV/AIDS drugs. These social evils hinder the quality life for many people. The story of creation should spur the church to take up its prophetic role in calling for a just world, a good world, where no one is discriminated against or lives in poverty. This was God's will for all life and people.

Given that the number one sponsor of HIV/AIDS is poverty, followed by gender inequalities, the church has to take a position on these issues. The story of creation is notable for holding that both men and women were created in God's image, hence equal; that they were both blessed and given the resources of the earth, hence they have leadership and decision making rights and powers. Poverty is against God's intention for human beings. The church can and should undertake to fight the poverty and gender inequalities that fuel the HIV/AIDS attack on life.

Song

See the Kingdom
You can get a poet to chant this song or choose another song

Solo: I have seen the kingdom,
Descending upon our mountains and hills;
I have seen its justice flooding our valleys and streets;
I have seen God in your eyes.

All: I have seen you,
I have seen your eyes, eyes like mine;
Looking out searching for the Kingdom;
I have seen God in your eyes, (2x)
God in your eyes.

Solo: I have heard the kingdom,
Ringing the melody of freedom upon our front yards;
Calling out, searching for the kingdom in our homes,
I heard the sound of God's justice in your laughter and voice;
I have heard God in your voice.

All: I have heard you,
I have heard your call, call like mine;
Calling out, calling for the kingdom;
I have heard God in your call; (2x)
God in your voice.
(By Musa W. Dube)

A Closing Prayer of Praise

Creator God, you are beautiful in your created world;
You are beautiful in the trees that swing and in the wind that blows;
You are beautiful in the stars that shine and in the sun that rises and sets;
You are beautiful in the animals that creep and roar;
You are beautiful in the faces of our families, friends--in all people;
We see your beauty in all the forms of creation;
The earth and the heavens tell of your beauty, love and goodness.
We thank you for the gift of life, for the sacred touch and spark in all life;
Help us to celebrate it, to live, to protect it, to maintain it;
Help us to be good custodians of life; to be good stewards of your resources;
Help us to fight against all the social injustices that mar the beauty of your creation;
Help us to fight HIV/AIDS and its plunder on life and the quality of life;
Creator God, grant us another day, another season, another year to life,
So we can live in praise of your loving touch and creative hand of life.
This we pray, in Jesus name. Amen

Symbols/objects/ideas: A new born baby, a basket of seeds, a pot with plant/s, flowing water, seeds, fresh assorted flowers, wall cloth depicting rainbow colors of God's creation, narration of local creation stories or proverbs, celebrative dances and songs of joy, etc.

By Musa W. Dube

LIFE

Sermon Text: Genesis 1-2

Introduction

HIV/AIDS is a fundamental negation of life. The absence of a known cure, poverty, sexism and stigma, have all coagulated to make life lonely and burdensome for the infected and affected. In some African cities, advertising signs indicate the price of affordable coffins, and death has become a common occurrence. Wailing, funeral processions and other practices associated with death are regular experiences in many African communities.

The creation story reaffirms life as proceeding from God. The text highlights God's active role in the creation of the world. Consequently, anything that threatens life is contrary to the will of God. HIV/AIDS threatens human existence and should be challenged. The vibrancy and beauty of the created order can be restored after HIV/AIDS has been overcome.

We Listen to the Word of God

Emphasize the fact that life has beginning in God's creative power. It is God who creates and affirms. The creation of humanity is also based on God's desire that humans may enjoy abundant life. However, God also commands humanity to observe a specific code of conduct, if this life is to be assured. In essence, the creation story captures the ideal condition where disease and death do not frustrate and terminate life. We need to keep life in God's intended goodness, namely where every relationship remains good. In such a God willed world, poverty, diseases, corruption, and the oppression of women and children should be countered, for they negate life as created by the creator.

We Apply the Word of God to Ourselves

WHAT CAN WE LEARN?
- God supports life;
- Humans have a special responsibility in nurturing life;
- All human being were created in God's image.

WHAT DO WE HAVE TO CONFESS?
- Not seeing HIV/AIDS as a challenge to a life, willed by God;
- Overlooking the vitality of life over death;
- Sitting in silence over poverty, the abuse of human rights and the environment.

WHAT CAN WE BE THANKFUL FOR?
- God's gift of life;
- Medical advancement in HIV/AIDS issues;
- The presence of God in all life forms.

We Apply the Word of God to the Congregation

Ask the congregation to reflect on the following issues:
How do factors like stigma, poverty, gender inequalities, etc. threaten God's promise of life?

- How does HIV/AIDS necessitate a rereading of being fruitful and multiplying?
- What can they do to ensure abundant life in HIV/AIDS contexts?

Conclusion: A Word on Society

God wills that humans should enjoy full lives. All systems that are oppressive, like patriarchy, neocolonialism and others that fuel HIV/AIDS should be resisted. Leaders at the various levels should therefore ensure that life is promoted and the forces of death are repelled.

Song

All the Earth Proclaim the Lord

(CLG Hymn Book, 102)

OR

Hakuna akaita saJesu
Hakuna akaita saye

Ndatsvaga tsvaga kwese kwese
Hakuna

(Popular chorus)

Prayer

Creator God, Maker of Heaven and Earth,
May all creation testify to your greatness.
Your breath sustains life,
It banishes disease, death and suffering.
Women and men, you created us in your image;
Our sustainer and enabler,
We praise and adore you;
We lift up your holy name;
We cry out for forgiveness;
For we have harmed your beautiful creation.
Dear God, we beseech you to allow us a new start,
As we celebrate the mystery of the created order.
Guide us and protect us through Jesus Christ. Amen

Poem

AFFIRMING LIFE AMIDST HIV/AIDS E. C.

    "Coffins for Sale" screams the sign

    "Abundant Life" screams the preacher

    Death stalks

    But Life beckons

    Tears everywhere

    Everywhere graves

    Somewhere the old rugged cross

    Offers an open invitation

    Poverty, sexism and stigma

    Authors of doom and gloom

    Love, sacrifice and solidarity

    Fountains of life eternal

    Created in Gods' image

    Proceeding from Gods' hands

    Humans shall prevail

    O HIV/AIDS: Where is your sting?

Suggested Objects/symbols/ideas: Water (life, potentiality); flowers (beauty of creation); green branches (vitality); stones (longevity).

                By Ezra Chitando

VIDA

Texto sugerido: Marcos 1:40-45

Introdução

Acreditar na cura quando se está gravemente doente, é algo cada vez mais raro na nossa sociedade. Nas cidades africanas é comum ver doentes mentais abandonados(as) pelos familiares a deambular pelas ruas. Alguns (as) deles (as) são apredejados (as), outros (as) atropelados (as) e são motivo de risota por parte de muita gente. As ruas estão cheias de crianças abandonadas. Nos hospitais também encontram-se doentes cujas famílas já não querem cuidar. Isso acontece porque as pessoas deixaram de acreditar na vida. Na era do HIV/SIDA, mesmo pessoas não doentes, não acreditam na vida. Isso faz com que o procedimento de muitos (as) seja pouco digno. A conclusão a que chegamos é de que, tal como o leproso do texto, nós também estamos infectados (as) e afectados (as) pelo HIV/SIDA, ou outras enfermidades, e deixamos de viver. Todavia, para continuarmos a viver, precisamos de ter fé. Devemos ir ter com Jesus e dizer-lhe: Limpa-nos, tira-nos o medo da morte. Precisamos de ser tocados (as) pela compaixão de Jesus para podermos ir ao encontro das pessoas que estão doentes e tocá-los (as). Temos que nos levantar e voltar à vida.

Vamos Escutar a Palavra de Deus

Leia o texto e sublinhe com um lápis as palavras mais importantes.

DETALHES
V 40-1:
➢ Novo Testamento conta muitos episódios de pessoas doentes marginalizadas pela sociedade que, tendo gritado, chorado, ajoelhado ou tocado Jesus, foram foram por Ele curadas. O leproso de Marcos, é um deles.

V 41-43:
➢ Jesus não aceita qualquer tipo de marginalização nem de estigmatização. Dá-nos uma lição, tocando, curando e ensinando aquilo que deve ser o procedimento de um crente.

VV. 44-45:
➢ testemunho do ex-leproso.

A Palavra de Deus Para Nós

QUE PODEMOS APRENDER?
• Que Jesus veio ao mundo para salvar a todos sem excepção.

QUE PODEMOS CONFESSAR?
• Que muitas vezes, por vergonha, escondemos as nossas doenças e as dos nossos familiares e acabamos por morrer.
• Que ainda temos dúvida de que a fé pode curar.

Pregamos a Lei de Deus: Deut 30:19

Canção
Escolha uma canção que celebra a vida

Oração
Santo, Santo, Santo é o teu nome. A paz, o amor e a justiça vem de ti. Que seria de nós sem Ti? Graças te damos porque nos amas. A Tua presença na nossa vida é uma dádiva inquestionável. Ajuda-nos Senhor a compreender o tipo de missão que nos deste. Só com esse conhecimento seremos capazes de dar testemunho sincero e, de fazer com que o teu Reino seja ensinado sem deturpações. Em nome de Jesus oramos. Amen

Por: Felicidade N. Cherinda

2. Compassion

If YOU DID IT TO THE LEAST OF THESE…YOU DID IT TO ME
Sermon Passage: Matthew 25:31-46

Call to Worship

Leader:	I am because we are.
All:	We are because I am.
Leader:	No person is an island.
All:	Our God is the triune God, the God with us.

Introduction

The HIV/AIDS epidemic has struck fear in our hearts. It is the fear of being infected with an incurable disease, the fear of suffering for a long time before one's death, the fear of dying and dying alone, the fear of coming out with one's health status and being rejected, the fear of facing one's shattered dreams, the fear of leaving behind young and growing children. Fear; fear everywhere. This fear has, in many ways brewed stigma and discrimination and the isolation of those who are infected and who are already sick. It has hindered the provision of quality care. It has hindered compassion just when it is needed most. Compassion is defined as the reaching out to those who are suffering, as entering of their places of pain, their brokenness and the active search for ways of changing of their situation. Compassion is transformative.

In the gospel of Luke 6:36, Jesus said, "Be compassionate as your Father is compassionate." Christ commands the church to be compassionate. In Matthew 25:31-46, Jesus makes perhaps the most compelling case for the Christian church to be compassionate. Jesus calls upon all his followers to see him in the faces of those who are hungry, thirsty, homeless, naked, sick and imprisoned. He identifies himself with them. Serving these or failing to serve them, is tantamount to doing it to Jesus. This passage calls us in the most compelling way to hear and feel the pains of Jesus in the faces and cries of sorrow of the infected and affected. We *must* be compassionate, if we count ourselves worthy to enter God's kingdom.

We Listen to the Word of God

Reading Matthew 25: 31-46

DETAILS OF THE TEXT
Verses 31-34:
- ➤ Note the setting: it is the judgment day, the second coming of Christ, and "All the nations will be gathered before him."
- ➤ "All nations" suggests that the criterion that will be applied at the judgment is expected for all people—it is not optional.
- ➤ Judgment day separates the good from the bad, sheep from goats, the right hand from the left hand. Some inherit God's kingdom. Some get sent to the eternal fire. What is the criterion?

Verses 35-36:
- ➤ The decision is based on having given food to the hungry; water to the thirsty; hospitality to strangers; clothes to the naked; care to the sick; a visit to the imprisoned. The criteria for inheriting the kingdom of God, is what one does to the underprivileged or marginalized.
- ➤ The criterion is compassion.
- ➤ Underline the verb "I was.... " that is, Jesus identifies himself with the hungry, thirsty, naked, sick, stranger, prisoners. You cannot separate Christ from these. (Luke 4:18-19)

Verses 37-41:
- ➤ Note that those who are commended for their compassion are surprised. They ask, "When was it that we saw you...?" The answer is "Truly I tell you, just as you did it to one of the least of these who are members of my family, you did it to me."
- ➤ Emphasize that "seeing Jesus" entails seeing the marginalized and taking action to meet their needs.
- ➤ Highlight that once more Jesus underlines his solidarity with the marginalized, he calls them "members of my family."
- ➤ Underline that Jesus says "just as you did it to...these... you did it to me."
  Jesus is one with the suffering, the marginalized. Our compassion to the marginalized, is service to Christ.
- ➤ Underline that in this passage, compassion is the only criterion given for inheriting the kingdom of God, thus underlining its centrality to Christian faith.
  See also Luke 16:19-31.
- ➤ Emphasize that compassion is about suffering with the suffering, but above all it is entering their situation order to change it—the hungry become fed, the thirsty get water, the homeless are welcomed, etc. Compassion, in other words, is transformative. It must challenge and seek to change the social structures that make people hungry, thirsty, homeless, sick, imprisoned, etc.

Verses 42-43:

➢ Highlight that, according to the text, those who are thrown "into the eternal fire prepared for the devil." Those who fail to inherit the kingdom of God, fail because of their lack of compassion. They failed to serve the needy—who are one with Christ. To fail the needy is to fail Christ.

Verse 44-46:

➢ This group is also surprised by the harsh judgment. They ask, "When was it that we saw you hungry, or thirsty, or a stranger, or naked, or sick, or in prison, and did not take care of you?" The answer is, "Just as you did not do it to one of the least of these, you did not do it to me."

➢ Underline that failure to be compassionate to those in need, is to fail Christ.

➢ Underline that in this story of judgment, there is no other criterion for inheriting the kingdom of God, only compassion is required (see also Luke 16:19-31). This underlines its centrality. Compassion is a must.

We Apply the Word of God to Ourselves

WHAT CAN WE LEARN?

• That compassion is not optional for Christians, it is a must;
• That being compassionate to the marginalized is being compassionate to Christ;
• That at the end compassion is the one and only expected criterion for measuring true Christian discipleship.
• That our compassion should be applied to all people, regardless of their religion, health status, race, ethnic, class, gender national or international status;
• That compassion must be practiced by both women and men.

WHAT DO WE HAVE TO CONFESS?

• We confess that we have not always been compassionate;
• We have not always seen compassion as central to our Christian faith;
• We have sometimes confused charity with compassion.

WHAT CAN WE BE THANKFUL FOR?

• That Christ calls us to be compassionate;
• That the ministry of Christ is an example of compassion;
• We all have an opportunity to begin and apply compassion.

WHAT CAN WE PRAY FOR?

• To practically represent the compassion Christ in the world;
• To live out compassion of Christ in the HIV/AIDS era.

We apply the Word of God to the Congregation

WHAT CAN WE BE?
- A compassionate church, Christian workers and citizens of God's world.

WHAT CAN WE DO?
Undertake programmatic acts of compassion to:
- Meet the needs of all the marginalized;
- Fight HIV/AIDS and its stigma.

Conclusion: A Word on Society

Society is laden with social injustice. Even though the creator God gave all people access to the earth's resources, there are many people who are hungry, thirsty, sick, naked and imprisoned. General society has become so used to living with injustice, and the church needs to remind society that God does not tolerate injustice. Through its concrete acts of compassion, the church should serve the marginalized as its service to Christ. With HIV/AIDS, which has been characterized by fear, stigma and discrimination, and which is fueled by poverty and gender inequality, the need to live out our Christian witness of compassion cannot be overstated. It is imperative.

Song

I Heard You
(Or, What a Friend we have in Jesus)

Solo:
I have heard your cry of pain;
I have heard your pumping heart, beating like mine;
Pushing hard, searching for the kingdom;
I have heard the cry of God's kingdom in your cry. (2x)

All:
I have heard you;
I have heard your cry, cry like mine;
Crying out, crying for the kingdom;
I have heard God in your cry; (2x)
God in your voice.

Solo:
I have felt the kingdom;
Touching my heart when your warm hand touched me;
I have felt the pain of God in your pain;
I have felt the joy of God in your joy. (2x)

All:
You have touched me;
You have touched my heart, with your heart;

Feeling out, feeling for the kingdom;
I have felt God in your touch; (2x)
God in your touch.

(By Musa W. Dube)

Closing: Responsive Prayer

Leader: Open our eyes Oh Lord,
All: So that we can see you in the faces of those who suffer from HIV/AIDS.
Leader: Open our hearts,
All: So we can feel the pains of all who suffer as your sorrow and suffering.
Leader: Open our ears,
All: So that we can hear the cry of the grieving as your cry.
Leader: Open our hands,
All: So we can serve and feed the orphans, widows and people living with HIV/AIDS (PLWHA's).
Leader: Open our feet,
All: So we can go and be with those who are in home-based care.
Leader: Open our minds,
All: So we can become prophetic to social injustice that fuels HIV/AIDS.

Commissioning

Go with the God of compassion.
Go with Emmanuel, the God With Us.
Go with the Comforter to liberate creation from oppression.
Go and heal God's people and world.

Suggested Objects/symbols/ideas: Pictures (of touching hands, holding hands, couples supporting each other, nurses and doctors with patients), tell the story of Nelson Mandela from a compassionate view, display Zimbabwean abstract stone carvings on interdependence or support, tell your own experience of receiving compassion.

By Musa W. Dube

OCASIÕES DIVERSAS
COMPAIXÂO
Texto sugerido: Lucas 13:10-17

Oração

Senhor, nosso Deus, eis-nos perante ti, cheios de alegria e de louvores. Estamos orgulhosos porque sabemos que nos criaste e nos amas. Ajude-nos na nossa caminhada, para nunca nos afastarmos da tua vontade, todos os dias da nossa vida. Amen

Introdução

O Evangelho de Lucas tem muitas passagens que não constam nos outros. Esta é uma delas. Nesta história, ao contrário do que geralmente acontece, Jesus, por iniciativa própria, interrompe o sermão para chamar e curar uma mulher que andava encurvada havia 18 anos. Não é por acaso que Jesus chama uma mulher. Naquele tempo e, ainda nos nossos dias, as mulheres são marginalizadas. São consideradas seres inferiores, incapazes, que só servem para agradar ao homem, dar-lhe filhos, tomar conta da casa e das machambas. Depois de curá-la , Jesus recorda aos presentes que ela também é filha de Abraão. Logo após a cura, a mulher louva a Deus. O principe da Sinagoga não gostou, e imediatamente fez conhecer a sua fúria dizendo que o Sábado não era dia para curar pessoas. Vendo isso, Jesus denunciou ali mesmo a falsidade e da sua pregação. Se as igrejas investissem um pouco nas mulheres, será que a situação não iria melhorar? Basta recordar que o HIV/SIDA só vai diminuir quando as mulheres se colocarem na vanguarda pelo seu combate. Jesus chamou o príncipe da Sinagoga de hipócrita porque escondia a sua falcidade no cumpimento da lei. Não é isso que acontece nas nossas igrejas?

Escutemos a Palavra de Deus

Leia o texto e sublinhe as palavras mais importantes.

DETALHES
VV. 10-13:
➢ Jesus pára de ensinar para curar uma mulher anónima.Essa mulher louva a Deus na Sinagoga.
V 14:
➢ Invocando a Lei, o príncipe da Sinagoga fica indignado com a atitude de Jesus.
VV. 15-16:
➢ Jesus denuncia a hiprocrisia do príncipe.
V 17:
➢ povo rejubila pelas obras de Jesus.

A Palavra de Deus para nós

QUE PODEMOS APRENDER?
- Que não existe nenhuma tarefa que pode nos impedir de socorrer aqueles que estão em perigo ou doentes.
- Que não devemos abandonar alguém só por estar doente há muito tempo.
- Que devemos denunciar as mentiras que são proferidas nos púlpitos.
- Que a igreja é para todos sem distinção de raça, sexo, cor da pele, etc.
- Que a Lei de Deus resume-se no mandamento que diz : Amarás ao teu próximo como a ti mesmo.

QUE TEMOS DE CONFESSAR?
- Que as nossas pregações, muitas vezes ofendem, acusam, expulsam e estigmatizam as pessoas.
- Que nos é difícil partilhar o que é nosso com doentes, principalmente os infectados pelo HIV/SIDA.
- Que na nossa pregação, O Reino de Deus está dividido.
- Que nas nossas igrejas continuamos a colocar as mulheres em segundo plano.

QUE DEVEMOS PEDIR NAS NOSSAS ORAÇÔES?
- Que Deus nos perdoe e ilumine os nossos corações para compeendermos cada vez melhor a sua vontade.

A Palavra de Deus para a Sociedade

- Que atitude tomam os líderes nos diversos escalões quando se pretende modificar algumas práticas nas nossas igrejas?
- Como reagem quando se pretende restaurar a dignidade de alguém que tinha sido afastado (a) por se considerar pecador (a) ou infectado (a) pelo HIV/SIDA?

PREGAMOS A LEI DE DEUS : Lc 4:18-19

CANÇÂO
Escolha uma canção apropriada para o momento

Oração
Senhor, tu és Deus único, que perdoa ao pecador, que conhece as suas dores, as suas fraquezas, o seu sofrimento. Agradecemos a tua presença incondicional na nossa vida. Afaste de nós o orgulho que nos impede de aceitar os (as) nossos (as) irmãos (ãs) na tua obra. Pedimos isto,em nome daquele que veio para que todos tenhamos vida em abundância, Jesus Cristo. Amen

Por: Felicidade N. Cherinda

3. Hope

HOPE: "PROPHESY TO THESE BONES"
Sermon Text: Ezekiel 37:1-13

Call to Worship

Do you not know?
Have you not heard?
The LORD is the everlasting God,
The Creator of the ends of the earth.
He will not grow tired or weary,
And his understanding no one can fathom.
He gives strength to the weary,
And increases the power of the weak.
Even youths grow tired and weary,
And young men stumble and fall;
But those who hope in the LORD
Will renew their strength.
They will soar on wings like eagles;
They will run and not grow weary,
They will walk and not be faint.

Song

Uya memeza uHezekiya. Uthi mathambo hlanganani (Ezekiel is calling out saying, 'Let the bones come together').

Introduction

Depicted clearly in this passage, is a situation of utter and complete hopelessness in which the Israelites find themselves. It is a situation of a long and hopeless exile. Such hopelessness is familiar for many in the so-called Third World. The twin ravages of poverty and the HIV/AIDS pandemic combine to create a situation of death and hopelessness. Such situations are seldom the focus of the world's regard. They are too ghastly to attract world attention. Indeed, even in the countries where HIV/AIDS is wiping out villages and cities, people would rather look away and not allow the chilling reality to confront them. Such looking away plays itself out in the stigma attached HIV/AIDS, and the common self-delusion that HIV/AIDS happens to others and not to oneself. The HIV/AIDS pandemic is a low valley in the history and lives of the peoples of the world. This is especially true for the peoples of Africa. But people prefer mountain tops not valleys. People prefer to look up at the mountain rather than down in the valley. So the prophet is 'driven' by the spirit to a valley. The prophet Ezekiel is driven by the spirit to a valley full of lifeless bones - a deliberately exaggerated selected mix of metaphors - is one with which many Africans have found connection and resonance. The setting is one in which the prophet Ezekiel is led to the valley of dry bones and engaged in a dueling conversation by God. God wishes to transform the valley of death into a valley of life and hope. The very space of death and hopelessness will and can be transformed.

103

We Listen to the Word of God

The passage may either be read or dramatized. If the dramatization route is taken, then a number of people may be asked to lie still on the stage dramatizing the dry bones. The prophet Ezekiel character will then be 'thrown into the scene' to symbolize being driven to the valley whereupon he will continue to use the dialogue words from the passage. There will be a voice-over to personify God and to enable the dialogue between God and Ezekiel. First, the bodies of people will move around vigorously, to indicate the coming together of the bones. But they will go dead and quiet again; "Until the voice will speak again, and the breath of life if breathed into them."

DETAILS OF THE TEXT
We have already remarked on the fact that Ezekiel is involuntarily driven to the valley. This might mean that such a place was not one he would have ordinarily chosen to go to. Ezekiel was 'forcibly removed' from his comfort zone and forced to go not the mountain top, but to a terrible valley. Once at the valley, Ezekiel was required not merely to look down or to observe at a distance. First he was made to descend into the valley, and then he was led back and forth among the bones. He saw and felt the bones at close range and he remarked that they were very dry. The dialogue between Ezekiel and God is an intriguing one. Completely non-committal and full of doubt, Ezekiel is led by the hand as it were, to do as he was told and to witness a miracle.

We Apply the Word of God

WHAT CAN WE LEARN?
- That there are valleys not far from where we live. These could be hospitals, orphanages of HIV/AIDS hospices, or informal settlements.
- It is important for us not to be judgmental, but to visit the valleys of HIV/AIDS devastation.
- That in life there are mountaintops as well as valleys.
- That God can change situations which look totally hopeless.
- That we must never give up hope even in the face of apparently insurmountable obstacles.

WHAT DO WE HAVE TO CONFESS?
- That we prefer the mountain tops and avoid the valleys in our own backyards.
- In the absence of a cure for HIV/AIDS and in the face of the combination of HIV/AIDS, poverty and gender violence, we have been tempted to give up all hope.
- We have not done enough to prevent HIV/AIDS and the subsequent spread of hopelessness.

WHAT CAN WE BE THANKFUL FOR?
- For the hope that God has planted in us;
- For both the valleys and the mountaintops in our lives;
- That no situation is beyond the intervention and redemption of God.

WHAT CAN WE PRAY FOR?
- We pray for hope;
- We pray that God may give us courage to visit the valleys;
- We pray that God will resurrect all the dry bones in the valleys.

We Apply the Word of God to the Congregation

WHAT CAN WE FEEL?
- We can feel touched by the depth of despair in our communities;
- We can feel compassion for those infected and affected by HIV/AIDS;
- We feel thankful that hope and resurrection are firm promises from God.

WHAT CAN WE BE?
- We can become ambassadors of hope;
- We can become fearless sojourners and visitors of the valleys of hopelessness;
- We can become counselors, prophets and ministers of those who live in the valleys of dry bones.

WHAT CAN WE DO?
- We can minister to those in despair.

Conclusion: A Word to Society

Whereas the medical and biological symptoms and effects of the HIV/AIDS epidemic are often highlighted, an equally important aspect of this epidemic is its ability to eat away the hope and sense of purpose of individuals and communities. In this sense the HIV/AIDS epidemic can turn a vibrant community (or individual) with a bright outlook on life, into a bag of bones without flesh and without breath. It is in killing hope that HIV/AIDS is at its most devastating. Here both those infected and affected are equalized. They all live without hope and without meaning. This is an important pastoral challenge for the church. The prerequisite for taking part in a ministry of hope and creation is to be fearless of valleys - even the valleys full of dry bones.

Prayer of Commitment
Prayer of Assisi

Song
Any appropriate Easter Sunday song may be sung.

Symbols/objects/ideas and commitments: The testimony of people living fruitfully with HIV/AIDS, candles etc.

By Tinyiko S. Maluleke

HOPE: REBUILDING AFRICA
Sermon Text: Ezra 1:1-11

Introduction

One of the greatest casualties in the HIV/AIDS epidemic in Africa is hope. As orphans, widows and widowers increase, a sense of helplessness has gripped the continent. Suffering, disease and death have bred pessimism and despair. As a result, hope has become a scarce commodity. It is important to regenerate hope within communities affected by HIV/AIDS. New prophets and leaders should be stirred up to engage in activities that prevent the spread of HIV and provide quality care to the infected. Despite the suffering caused by the epidemic, communities of faith need to be empowered to look forward to the future and rejoice in hope.

We listen to the Word of God

In interpreting this text, emphasize the centrality of a sense of call and mission in undertaking the project of rebuilding the temple. This same conviction is required if HIV/AIDS is to be tackled in Africa. Also, highlight the different social and religious groups that were spurred into action. Although financial resources were crucial to the project, human and spiritual resources were equally vital.

We apply the Word of God to Ourselves

WHAT CAN WE LEARN?
- The need to have our spirits stirred up in the fight against HIV/AIDS.
- Reconstruction is still possible after devastation and war.
- Various social groups and actors should contribute in meeting the HIV/AIDS challenge.
- The church needs to take up leadership and to network with various stakeholders in the HIV/AIDS fight.

WHAT DO WE HAVE TO CONFESS?
- Hardening our spirits when the call to participate in fighting HIV/AIDS is made;
- Failing to provide adequate resources for awareness, prevention and care;
- Failure to provide leadership and to network with various stakeholders.

WHAT CAN WE BE THANKFUL FOR?
- Some individuals have prophetically taken up the struggle against HIV/AIDS.
- For those who have generously donated their valuable energy, time and financial resources.

WHAT CAN WE PRAY FOR?
- That more people be stirred up to confront HIV/AIDS;
- For the church to respond programmatically in the HIV/AIDS struggle.

We apply the Word of God to the Congregation

The preacher should underline the fact that African societies devastated by HIV/AIDS are similar to the temple in Jerusalem when it was destroyed. There is an urgent need for new visionaries to become agents of hope and reconstruction.

Ask members what they are doing or giving to the struggle against HIV/AIDS.
Indicate that the need to proclaim a vision of renewal is an urgent one in Africa.

Conclusion: A Word on Society

The rebuilding of the temple became possible through a prophetic vision and the mobilization of resources. Similarly, the HIV/AIDS challenge should inspire new prophets and different social groups to actively encounter it. Thus, every one should contribute to the fight and to inspire hope.

Song

We shall overcome, (3x) some day
O deep in my heart, I do believe, we shall overcome some day.
(CLG Hymn Book, No. 41)

Or

Jesu wedu, Jesu wedu inhamba one (x3)
Kana tasvika pane zvakaoma (x3)

(Popular chorus)

Prayer

One: Holy God, hear our cry.
All: If we are without hope,
Weighed down and affected by HIV/AIDS,
Prone to stigma and discrimination,
Hear us and help us.
One: Holy Creator, hear our cry.
All: When we ignore visions to combat HIV/AIDS,
Pass by widows and orphans,
Preach doom and destruction,
Hear us and help us.
One: Listen now to the message of hope,
After the darkest night the moon shines the brightest,
Disease and pain shall be banished,
Stigma and discrimination shall be overcome.
All: All praise and honor be yours!
God of hope, love and mercy,
The Spirit is with us!   Amen

Suggested Objects/symbols/ideas: Pictures of rebuilt cities, tell a story about African nations and their efforts to rebuild after years of war and destruction. You can use the story of your own country.
By Ezra Chitando

HOPE: DO NOT FEAR; ONLY BELIEVE
Sermon Text: Mark 5:21-43

Prayer

Leader: In the power of the creative Spirit of God, we come together to light a candle of hope in the hearts of all the people who are faced with hopeless situations. We are God's instruments to bring hope. Amen

Song

Siyahamb' ekukhanyeni kwe Nkos'// (We are walking in the light of God)
Siyahamb' ekukhanyeni kwe Nkos'// (We are walking in the light of God) (2x)
Siyahamba hamba// (We are walking, walking)
Siyahamba, Oh // (We are walking, Oh)
Siyahamb' ekukhanyeni kwe Nkosi // (We are walking in the light of God) (2x)

(Thuma Mina, No. 107)

Introduction

HIV is considered a terminal illness. Yet as Archbishop Desmond Tutu, a South African Black Theologian who had cancer said, 'Life is a terminal illness'. Is can be assumed that his statement was said to emphasize the temporary nature of life for everyone. As is often stated by Canon Gideon Byamugisha, a Ugandan HIV/AIDS activist, HIV is manageable. In the West, people live longer even when they have HIV, because of the availability of drugs at affordable prices. The drugs make HIV lay dormant in the body for a very long time. In Africa, the majority of the people cannot afford such drugs. Hope is one of the major sources of strength for the majority of the people as they survive on a daily basis. Africa is working urgently to seek solutions for HIV/AIDS for herself.

We Listen to the Word of God

Read or dramatize the text of Mark 5: 21-43

Chapter 5 is about Jesus restoring people's lives. Jesus restored a man who was possessed by demons to normal life. Jesus restored the life of Jairus' daughter from death. Jesus restored the health of a woman who had an issue of blood for twelve years.

DETAILS OF THE TEXT

Jairus was one of the rulers in the Synagogue. He went out to look for Jesus because his daughter was sick. Jesus went to Jairus' home to heal his daughter, but was delayed by another person who also needed help. While on the way to his house, Jairus received a message that his daughter was dead. Jesus encouraged him to continue trusting for the healing of his daughter. When they reached his home, Jesus commanded Jairus' daughter to wake up, which she did. The woman who had an issue of blood, had suffered for twelve years. In the processes of looking for treatment, she lost all her money. Her status made her impure and so she could not be in the midst of people. The disease itself made her weak and therefore vulnerable to other infections.

108

Most likely she could not keep a husband with her condition. She had faith that if she touched Jesus' clothes she would be healed, which she did. Jesus noticed her touch of faith and asked her to own up, which she did. Jesus praised her for her faith and she was healed.

We apply the Word of God to Ourselves

WHAT CAN WE LEARN?
- Like Jairus, men can play a significant role in caring for the sick, especially now when a lot of people have HIV/AIDS.
- The knowledge that Jesus is always available and willing to help. Jesus was a man of social status, but had time to go with Jairus to his house.
- Jesus was willing to be interrupted by the woman. This is important because sometimes we are so busy, to the extent that we do not hear people's cries for help.
- Jesus broke cultural taboos by speaking to this woman.
- When people touch us (seek our help) we loose power. This is particularly true for caregivers of AIDS patients.
- Jesus saw through Jairus to the girl child, who was a dispensable member of the society.
- The young girl was willing to hear the voice of Jesus. Young people need to be willing to hear the Word of God.
- There are many types of healings. Healing is not only physical. It can be spiritual, social, emotional, or even go beyond death (as far as God is concerned, there are other ways of being).

WHAT DO WE HAVE TO CONFESS?
- We have hindered some people from acting according to their faith, because of cultural beliefs and practices.
- Fathers have sometimes not contributed to taking care of the sick children.
- We have made ourselves too important, so that it is difficult for other people to seek our help.
- We have refused to be interrupted by needy people.
- Sometimes we do not listen to the needs of others, because we are loosing a lot of energy and we do not take notice.
- We have failed to hear the Word of God speaking to us.
- We have failed to see other forms of healing, because we concentrate on physical healing.

WHAT CAN WE BE THANKFUL FOR?
- The knowledge that God wants us to act according to our faith;
- That faith in God frees us from cultural restrictions;
- That there is hope even in the face of death.

WHAT CAN WE PRAY FOR?
- That we should exercise our faith at all times;
- There should be more fathers who are willing to help to give care for the sick;
- That we should be attentive to the voice of God all the time, so that we are able to know who needs our help, and how God wants us to help.

We Apply the Word of God to the Congregation

WHAT CAN WE FEEL?
- Repentant that we have been too busy to listen to those in need;
- Sorry for the mothers who work so hard to give care for the sick;
- Happy that there are fathers who help with giving care for the sick;
- Sad that cultural taboos make is difficult for us to love some people as Christ has shown us by example;
- Happy that death does not have the last word, Jesus does.

WHAT CAN WE BE?
- A community that helps each other in times of need;
- A healing community for people who are seeking any type of healing;
- A community that calls our children from death to life.

WHAT CAN WE DO?
- Hold seminars to teach the congregation about cultural practices that hinder us from helping those who are in need;
- Practice healing ministries for the various human needs;
- Take time for group or personal retreats to recharge our spiritual levels;
- Offer help to caregivers of AIDS patients, so that they too can take time off to recharge themselves;
- Offer counseling sessions for caregivers of terminally ill patients;
- Train our men to become caregivers.

Conclusion: A Word on Society

Care giving is an essential ministry and is should be recognized as such. Traditionally, care giving, especially for the sick, is considered to be a woman's job. HIV/AIDS has increased the burden of care giving. Most women find is difficult to cope by themselves. The story of Jairus challenges the concept that care giving of the sick is for women only, and highlights the contribution of fathers. It demands a societal change to the role of the father in care giving. The idea of sharing the role of care giving should be done out of love for the other, by recognizing that women are over stretched.

Hope is what life is all about. We are surrounded by death as a result of various situations. We have hope for restoration, sometimes experienced in this world and at other times, in the next world. That is the message of Christianity. As Paul says, "And we rejoice in the hope of the glory of God. Not only so, but we also rejoice in our suffering, because we know that suffering produces perseverance; perseverance, character; and character, hope. And hope does not disappoint us, because, God has poured out his love into our hearts by the Holy Spirit, whom he has given us." (Romans 5:2b-5)

Responsive Prayer

Leader: God of mercy, we recognize that the church of Jesus Christ has AIDS;

All: God of Love, we recognize you as the one who heals us;

Leader: God our Creator, we acknowledge the various ways that you heal your church.

All: God our Wisdom, open our eyes to see your many ways of healing;

Leader: God of Compassion, we see you taking time for the least of the society to bring them healing;

All: God our teacher, give us the courage to follow your foot-steps and bring healing to all people in our society;

Leader: We seek your forgiveness where we have failed you;

All: We receive your forgiveness as we go out to bring healing to your people through the power of the Holy Spirit. In Jesus' name, Amen.

Song (Chichewa)

Leader: Moyo wanga // (My life)

All: Moyo wanga umafuna Yesu // (My life wants Jesus) (4x)

Leader: Ndikadwala // (When I am sick)

All: Ndikadwala amandichilitsa // (When I am sick God heals me)

Leader: Ndikasowa // (When I am in need)

All: Ndikasowa amandipatsa // (When I am in need God gives me)

Leader: Ndikakhumudwa // (When I am discouraged)

All: Ndikakhumudwa amandilimbitsa // (When I am discouraged God makes me strong)

Leader: Moyo wanga // (My life)

All: Moyo wanga umakonda Yesu // (My life loves Jesus)

(A Malawian Community Song)

Benediction

Go in peace and with God to bring encouragement to the hopeless.

Objects/symbols/ideas: Testimonies from fathers who take their share in care giving for family members, people who have received different forms of healing from God, candles, doves, musical instruments.

By Isabel Apawo Phiri

4. Repentance

Sermon Text: Luke 18:9-14

Introduction

Before we look at the parable that Jesus gave, I want to offer you a modern day parable. There is a preacher in Gaborone, whose preaching draws many people to his congregation. He is by no means a modest man, he is always dressed with the latest designer suits and drives in flashy cars. On this occasion, he preaches on his favorite subject, fornication. He speaks with gusto and anger, declaring how those who have children outside marriage, the homosexuals and people living with HIV/AIDS, will be condemned to eternal damnation. As he preaches one of the people sitting in the congregation is HIV positive. She came with a friend, now she is cringing with shame as the preacher bellows away and she is regretting that she had come.

We Listen to the Word of God

DETAILS OF THE TEXT

Jesus tells a story of two characters with very contrasting attitudes to prayer. The first character is self-assured and exhibits a sense of spiritual pomp. He catalogues his deeds; he gives money regularly to the temple, prays a lot and is obviously an important person in society. He brags about this, and in fact uses this to denounce those who, in his opinion, do not match up to his piety. The other person is very humble and conscious of his shortcomings. He is remorseful for his sins and begs for mercy from God.

We Apply the Word of God to Ourselves and the Congregation

Who shall we say is represented by these two people in our communities today? Are there any connections between Jesus' parable and the modern parable in our introduction? It would help to compare the two, identify the common issues, as well as the differences in these two parables.

WHAT CAN WE LEARN?

Many people who suffer from HIV/AIDS have been verbally battered and assaulted by religious purists. They have not been allowed space within the church to express their remorse, like the tax collector, and therefore experience some healing. The Church needs to repent of the self-righteous attitude of the Pharisee, in order to become a community of healing and acceptance.

In Catholic churches, the ministry of repentance is taken seriously, because space is created for people to come to confession. It is important for the church to be a place where people are permitted to come to confession. It is important for the church to be a place where people are permitted to come in penitence before God, to pour out their emotions, bruised hearts and guilt for the sins they have committed. In the church, we should not just be allowed space to offer penitence, but to be assured of the love of Christ through absolution. Such a space, however, cannot exist if the church poses as a community of religious purity rather than one of love.

WHAT CAN WE CONFESS?
- Like the Pharisee and the preacher in the introduction, we are self-righteous;
- We make people 'small' through our sermons and prayers.

WHAT CAN WE BE THANKFUL FOR?
- The Church which is a 'school of sinners';
- The many humble pastors in the church who draw people to Christ through their ministry;
- The ministry of repentance and confession in the church.

WHAT CAN WE PRAY FOR?
(*Prayer of confession*):
Dear God, our creator, we come before you asking for your mercy. We have sinned against you and have forgotten your grace towards us. We have failed to be loving and accepting to those we live with. We often wrong the little ones among us through our arrogance. Forgive us our sins and restore us to fellowship with each other and with you. Amen

Song

Spirit of the living God,
Fall afresh on me.
Spirit of the living God,
Fall afresh on me.
Break me, melt me,
Mould me, fill me.
Spirit of the living Lord,
Fall afresh on me.
(Anonymous)

The Lord's Prayer

By all.

Suggested objects: The worship leaders could put up a small tree up front or in the middle (depending on the arrangement of the congregation), and upon this tree, people could pin up their prayers of confession. Another way could be to put the prayers in a bin and 'burn the sins' in front of the congregation

By Moiseraele P. Dibeela

5. Forgiveness

Sermon Text: Luke: 7:36-50

Introduction

One community building activity that is universal is having a meal together. It might be an ordinary meal, a wedding celebration, a funeral, communal work, a birthday party or any other party. Stories are heard that those who are HIV positive are being isolated from the fellowship table and made to eat by themselves for fear of being infected.

Jesus was invited to one of those dinners by a Pharisee. Let us take note that the main players in this episode are Simon, the host who is a Pharisee; Jesus, one of the guests; a nameless sinful woman who invites herself to the dinner; and other guests. It is the woman's action that prompts this little sermon on forgiveness given by Jesus.

We Listen to the Word of God

DETAILS OF THE TEXT
➢ What does the woman do? She brings with her an alabaster jar of perfume, stands at the feet of Jesus weeping, her tears wets his feet and she wipes them dry with her hair and pours perfume on them. Ask the congregation the following questions: Is this acceptable behavior? What was she communicating through these actions?

➢ Let us take note of the reaction of Simon, the Pharisee and host. Simon disapproves of the action and thinks it does not reflect well on the reputation of Jesus. Simon reproves Jesus for allowing himself to be touched by a sinful woman. Jesus risked being contaminated by her sinfulness. Simon did not verbalize his disapproval, but something about his body language communicated it and Jesus noticed.

➢ Let us take note of Jesus' own reaction. Jesus tells a parable using his proven teaching method. Ask the congregation the following questions: Who are the characters in the story? What is the problem? How is it resolved?

➢ Jesus asked Simon, "Which of them loved him more?" Simon answered, "I suppose the one who had the bigger debt." Jesus agreed with him.

➢ Now let us take note of Jesus' own attitude to the incident of the sinful woman. He contrasts Simon's behavior with that of the woman. Who comes out well and vindicated? Who comes out worse and condemned? Jesus has turned the tables. He stands not only as prophet, but a judge between Simon and the sinful woman. He is not only judge, but also the God who forgives sin and gives peace.

➢ The woman left liberated from the curse of her sinfulness, and ushered into the peace of God.

We Apply the Word of God to Ourselves and the Congregation

WHAT CAN WE LEARN?
- Ask the congregation to identify the main characters in the story;
- Ask the congregation to describe the main characters and say why they are found there;
- Why does Jesus use parables/stories in his teaching?
- The dynamics of the process of forgiveness;
- Jesus appreciation of the things the woman has done and how he met her need and blessed her with wholesomeness.

WHAT CAN WE CONFESS?
- Failure to do for others the common every day courtesies, as a sign of love and respect;
- Discrimination of women on the basis of gender;
- Condemning others without understanding them or their actions;
- Stigmatizing and discriminating people living with HIV/AIDS (PLHWA);
- Failure to minister to sex workers.

WHAT CAN WE PRAY FOR?
- For greater humility and a listening ear;
- For inclusive fellowship, especially for the poor, those who are HIV positive, sex workers and women;
- Forgiveness.

WHAT CAN WE FEEL?
- Explore with the congregation the feelings that this story generates and ask them why they experience those feelings.

WHAT CAN WE BE?
- An accepting and compassionate people of God;
- A forgiving and loving community-in-communion;
- An active community that practically seeks to empower women, PLWHA's and sex workers.

WHAT CAN WE DO?
- Show compassion;
- Meet the needs of the socially marginalized;
- Set up a support group for PLWHA's in the church;
- Begin programs for women's empowerment;
- Begin alternative income generating programs for sex workers.

We Apply the Word of God to the Congregation and Society

- How may pastors and even ordinary Christians would have tolerated what Jesus tolerated from the woman?
- Between Jesus and Simon, with whom would you have naturally identified with, in their reaction to the woman's actions?
- The Churches need to be sensitive to people's material and spiritual needs in order to minister to them adequately, instead of being judgmental.
- Love covers a multitude of sins. The issue is not the enormity of our sins, but the greatness of God's love and our response to it. Love never condemns. It rejoices when people finally find forgiveness and peace.
- This story challenges our theology of, and attitudes towards, sin and sinners. How ought we to think about sin and sinners in the light of God's love?
- The issue of the debt burden highlighted during the Millennium is still an issue for many poor countries. Is there something that lending institutions can learn from this story?

Song

God forgave my sins in Jesus' name,
I've been born again, in Jesus' name;
And in Jesus name, I come to you,
To share my life as he taught me to.

He said, freely, freely, you have received,
Freely, freely give.
God in my name and because you believe,
Others will know that I live.

Prayer: Response to a Litany of Confession

"Forgive us our trespasses as we forgive those who have trespassed against us."
Your sins are forgiven. Go in peace.

Suggested Objects/symbols/ideas: Crosses, flowers, gifts of food or cloth, drawing of a handshake or a hug, calabash of water, loosed chain or rope, perfume, sweet smelling oil.

By Augustine C. Musopule

6. Love

Sermon Text: I Corinthians 13:1-13

Introduction

Love in not only a language universal, but it is also a universal civilization. The culture of love expresses itself in the pleasure of loving. This is what the world needs and longs for, and yet what it lacks. This is what the world desires, but also that it misses. The world talks and sings about love a lot, but greatly misunderstands it. Our sense of love is conditional, functional and has strings attached, it is never free and spontaneous. The love that we are talking about in this text is very different from what we are used to. It was called *agape* in Greek, and means the invincible goodwill, or simply the "in-spite-of" kind of love. Paul calls it "the most excellent way." It is a spiritual gift. It is poured in the believer's heart by the Holy Spirit (Romans 5:5). It is foundational and also fundamental as the greatest commandment. It is the meaning of life, since we are created in the image of God whose very life and nature is love (I John 4:8). God's means of relating to the world is primarily one of love. We are created out of love, through love, with love and for love. God's justice is a consequence of God's love and not the other way round. In these days of HIV/AIDS, we need lots of love for God, for one another and for ourselves. Only love can give us the hope we need and only love can sustain our faith. Only love can help us to prevent HIV/AIDS and to provide care. It is love that makes us communities of compassion, and not those who stigmatize and discriminate those who are living with the disease.

We Listen to the Word of God

Read Mark 12:28-31 and John 13:34-35. This should help to set the context for our text. It might also be good to start reading the text from I Corinthians 12:27, so as to relate it to the church's corporate life. Love is presented in verse 31 as the greater gift and the most excellent way.

DETAILS OF THE TEXT

Verse 1-3:

➢ Love is contrasted with some other spiritual gifts. What is the evaluation when love is lacking? Without love, all other gifts lack value for God and for other people.

Verse 4-8a:

➢ We are presented with the character or nature of love. This serves as our benchmark to see how we are measuring up in our own humanness. Ask each to substitute their name for love to see if they measure up to the greatest commandment.

Verse 8b-10:

➢ Love's enduring quality is contrasted with prophecies and knowledge that have a limited duration and function. While these are powerful means for our security and salvation, they are imperfect.

117

Verse 11-12:

➢ Love is a sign of spiritual maturity. We grow spiritually and that growth is properly marked by love and not other spiritual gifts. The mark of a person filled by the Holy Spirit is love.

Verse 13:

➢ Presents three pillars of life: Faith, Hope and Love. Even among these, love is the greatest.

We Apply the Word to Ourselves and the Congregation

WHAT CAN WE LEARN?
- While other gifts are important for the corporate life of the church, it is love which is foundational. It is the hallmark of Christian living.
- The nature of love and that we need to excel in it.
- That prophecies and knowledge are imperfect or unreliable.
- We need to mature in our knowledge and practice of love.
- There are three champions in life: Faith, Hope, and Love, but the greatest of these is Love.

WHAT CAN WE CONFESS?
- Lifting other gifts above love, for instance speaking in tongues and healing miracles;
- Not maturing in our loving;
- Not obeying the commandment to love others as ourselves;
- Not measuring up to the true nature of love in our families, churches and community;
- That we have failed to love those who are HIV positive and that HIV/AIDS stigma and discrimination is sin before God.

WHAT CAN WE BE THANKFUL FOR?
- That in spite of the confusion over what love is, we can experience some measure of loving;
- That God is the inexhaustible source of genuine loving;
- That we can mature in love.

WHAT CAN WE PRAY FOR?
- The manifestation of love in the family of God;
- The ability to love those who are HIV positive or suffering from AIDS.

WHAT CAN WE FEEL?
- Love for God and for our neighbors;
- Love for self;
- Love for the world, so as to intercede for it;
- Compassion toward those who are suffering from AIDS.

WHAT CAN WE BE?
- People overflowing with love;
- People with compassion.

WHAT CAN WE DO?
- Reach out to orphans with love;
- Form support group those who are sick due to HIV/AIDS;
- Engage in an awareness campaign;
- Teach what it means to love and how to love genuinely;
- Reach out to widows with love.

We Apply the Word to the Congregation and Society

Just listen to any FM station, and you are bound to hear melancholic music about some aspect of love. Love seems to be the universal language. It is longed for and most missed. While we believe that love is the answer, more often than not, we do not know how to express it adequately. We often have wrong ideas about love, and we use the word to trap others in our greed and self-centredness. Genuine love is other-centred and seeks to serve the other, rather than self. While we talk a lot about love in the churches, there is little practice to show that we are serious. Love has to be our sense of being the church in the world, otherwise we are not the church. Since genuine love is a gift of the Holy Spirit, it is found nowhere in the world except in the church. Since it is a gift, it can only be offered to others as a gift. If we are going to be of any service to those who are HIV positive, we have to be first and foremost servants and prisoners of love.

Poem: "Love is Acting Justly"

Should we do our work together in love?
We are bound to succeed.
Jesus our Lord has commanded,
Love one another.
Love is to act justly,
Again I say,
Love is to act justly.
Words only prove inadequate
To remove bitterness;
To deal with silent in-fights
In our fellowship.

The surprise comes
While there is cooperation among us.
Attracting admiration from onlookers,
And yet silent wars continue to destroy our fellowship.

When wrong is done,
It is justified as right,
Making the wrong worse.
We know not how to do it better,

However, the truth is plain,
Satan has taken advantage of us
By stealing our ability to discern.
Love is to act justly,
Again I say,
Love is to act justly.
Words only prove inadequate
To remove the bitterness
To deal with silent in-fights
In our fellowship.

(Adapted from a song by Kufalitsa Uthenga Choir, Chongoni, Malawi)

Prayer: A Litany of Love

Leader:	Love is patient;
Congregation:	Patient God, you are always patient with us, teach us also to be patient with one another.
Leader:	Love is kind;
Congregation:	Kind God, you are always kind to us, teach us to be kind to one another.
Leader:	Love does not envy;
Congregation:	We confess that envy destroys our relationships daily. God who is not envious, teach us to appreciate one another.
Leader:	Love does not boast and it is not proud;
Congregation:	We confess our pride. Oh God, who shows your love in humility, teach us to offer humble service to one another.
Leader:	Love is not rude and self-seeking;
Congregation:	Good Lord, we confess that we are often rude to one another and also self-centred. Forgive us for the sake of Jesus Christ and make us new.
Leader:	Love is not easily angered and keeps no record of wrong;
Congregation:	We confess that often we keep records of wrong and are not able to reconcile ourselves to one another and to you. God, show us the futility of keeping such records, and the need to forgive and to forgive ourselves.
Leader:	Love does not delight in evil, but rejoices in the truth;
Congregation:	Help us Good Lord to delight in that which is good and true.
Leader:	Love always protects, trusts, hopes and always perseveres;
Congregation:	Help us Good Lord to experience this kind of love from you and others. May we always protect the orphans, the widows, and those suffering from HIV/AIDS discrimination and stigma, for the love of Jesus Christ.
Leader:	Love never fails;
Congregation:	Good Lord, we often experience failure with our types of love. Grant us your kind of love, so as to succeed in our loving endeavours. Amen

Suggested Objects/symbols/ideas: The cross, food, drink, water, towel, ring, love songs, kanga or kitenge cloth, a rose or some other item that expresses love and care.

By Augustine C. Mosupole

7. Fear and Desperation

Sermon Text: II Kings 6:24-30

Leader: We gather in the name of our Creator, who did not give us a spirit of fear, but of power, love and a sound mind. We join hands to work together towards the healing of our communities from injustice.

All: God is calling us to a ministry of reconciliation and peace.

Song (Chichewa)

Muzinthu zonse, zonse, zones // (In all things)
Muzinthu zonse Mulungu alemekezeke // (In all things God must be praised) (2x)

Akakhalapo // (When God is there) (2x)
Chigonjetso chilipompo//(Victory is there) (2x)
(A Malawian Community Song)

Introduction

History has shown us that war destroys life and hope. It dehumanizes people by making the victims of war live in fear and desperation. This is because the results of war are economic, health, political and gender-based injustice. War breeds insecurity, displacement of people, anger, selfishness, despair, and oppression of the poor and the marginalized. In recent times, research has shown that war promotes gender violence and the spread of HIV/AIDS. This is primarily because war destroys, and can bring every social welfare institution to a standstill: families, health, education and government systems come to a standstill, while money is ploughed into killing. War destroys life, and tramples down on the most valuable aspects of being. Even those who survive have been adversely affected. In such a context, epidemics can only rocket, and HIV/AIDS surely does.

In the Western media, the African people are presented as constantly fighting among themselves. It is a very bad image for all of us. We need to remind ourselves that there are many African countries where there is peace. We also have to thank God that African politicians are working hard to solve their own problems. We also have to remind ourselves that there are wars in many different parts of the world. They are a result of the sinful nature of humanity. But here is a ghastly truth: in the HIV/AIDS era, more people are killed by this plague than by war!! About five thousand people die a day of HIV/AIDS. What does such a huge attack on life do to our humanity—our spirits and our minds? What kind of fear and desperation is likely to arise? The passage that we are going to read is an example of the destructive nature of war, and how it can dehumanize those who live in it.

We Listen to the Word of God

The leader or a member of the congregation can read the text of II Kings 6:24-30, or a group can mime or dramatize the story.

The story is about what happens in a city that has been involved in war.

DETAILS OF THE TEXT
- ➢ Samaria was surrounded by the army of Aram for a long time.
- ➢ The people of Samaria lived in fear and were not able to trade with the people outside the city, and there was famine in the land.
- ➢ Due to famine, people started eating things which were considered unclean.
- ➢ The people became desperate to the point that useless things like a donkey's head were selling expensively.
- ➢ Women were particularly affected by the famine to the point of eating their own children.
- ➢ It took the desperate action of the two women and the testimony of one to move the king of Israel to begin to do something about it.

We Apply the Word of God to Ourselves

WHAT CAN WE LEARN?
- That war dehumanizes people. Therefore, we should not take life for granted. We should appreciate all the good things that we have, because in times of war those things are not easily available.
- That women in particular suffer more from war, because a majority are poor, and cannot afford to buy food in times of famine and war.
- That we should always work towards reconciliation to avoid war regardless the cost. We should also protect the environment and preserve food for hard times.
- That we should pray and help people who are affected by war and famine.
- That HIV/AIDS brings fear and desperation in people, just as war and famine.
- That leaders do not suffer from war, famine and HIV/AIDS, in the same way as ordinary people.

WHAT CAN WE CONFESS?
- Not supporting peace efforts with action to avert war, when countries are at loggerheads.
- Not supporting communities and countries affected by war, famine and HIV/AIDS.
- Not paying special attention to the suffering of women and children as a result of war.
- Not conscientising our political leaders to act quickly on behalf of the poor.
- Not allowing situations to push us to desperation and a life of fear.

WHAT CAN WE BE THANKFUL FOR?
- That God has promised us that God will never leave us or forsake us. Therefore, even in times of war, famine and HIV/AIDS, God is with us.
- That God did not give us a spirit of fear, but of power, love and a sound mind. Therefore, even during hard times, we have the power to change the way we respond to situations.

WHAT CAN WE PRAY FOR?
- For justice to prevail on earth.
- Reconciliation for countries and communities that are in conflict.
- For those who are living in situations of fear and desperation due to war, famine and HIV/AIDS and that solutions to their problems be found.
- In particular for women who suffer from gender violence in times of war, famine and HIV/AIDS.
- Our political leaders to be sensitive to the needs of their people.

We Apply the Word of God to the Congregation

WHAT CAN WE FEEL?
- Sorry for people who are living in conditions that are dehumanizing.
- Sad that our silence has led to the death of innocent people.
- Happy that God has given us power to lead change in our communities.

WHAT CAN WE BE?
- A community that works together to raise funds to support people who are suffering as a result of war, famine and HIV/AIDS.
- A community that is up to date with world events, so that our prayers and actions are informed.
- A community that support peace action.
- People who bring messages of hope to people who live in fear and desperation.

WHAT CAN WE DO?
- Raise funds to support people affected by war, famine and HIV/AIDS.
- Pray for people affected with famine, war and HIV/AIDS.
- Mobilize people to support peace efforts.
- Teach people who are living in fear and desperation, the promises of God.

Conclusion: A Word on Society

HIV/AIDS, like war, has struck fear and desperation in the hearts of many. The meaning of life is lost. The act of trying to hold on to it indicates dire desperation. This is clear in the rape of the girl child and of infants, by adult male strangers and relatives in attempt to cleanse themselves of HIV/AIDS. It is attested by some turning to bestiality, in fear of getting infected by human beings. It is also attested to by reports of some ignorantly turning to homosexuality, thinking it will be safer sex than heterosexuality (not surprising given the great silence concerning homosexuality in African communities). It is attested to by the general rise of rape. In short, any people who are under fear and desperation, can easily loose their humanity in attempt to survive.

The Christian community is called by God to become a light of hope in society. In times of fear and desperation, the Christians need to share Jesus' message of peace with the society. Christians should be seen to behave in a manner that is in line with God's message of peace and reconciliation. Therefore, what we say and do should be the same. The Creator God has given us the power to effect change in our communities. No human deserves to live with injustice. It is God's will that there should be justice for all humanity. There is no situation that we cannot change when we act in solidarity with the power that God has given us.

Song (Chichewa)

Mulungu angathe, angathe, angathe // (God is able)
Mulungu angathe salephera // (God is able, God does not fail)
Iye ndiye Alepha Omega // (God is Alpha and Omega)
Oyamba, Otsiliza // (The beginning and the end)
Wachipulumutso chamoyo wanga // (God is the saviour of my life)
Mulungu angathe salephera.// (God is able, God does not fail)
(A Popular Malawian Song)

Prayer

By all;

We thank you Creator God, for empowering each one of us with your Holy Spirit to effect change. When Jesus was on earth, he taught us not to live in fear and desperation. Even where there is suffering, you are there and you have a plan for your people. Your plan is good and brings life in abundance. You want to see justice on earth. You want us to be your instruments on earth to bring peace and justice. Give us courage to do what we know is right. In Jesus' name, Amen

Benediction

May you always stand for peace, justice and love in the name of Jesus.

Object/symbols/ideas: Candles and musical instruments.

By Isabel Apawo Phiri

8. Stigma and Discrimination

STIGMA
Sermon Text: Job 3:1-26

Introduction

Stigma is a condition that causes one to be shunned, discriminated against and even persecuted, for perceived moral, ethnical, gender, health, economic, physical, religious, class or social impropriety. The condition is seen either as a threat to the majority or powerful of a community; for instance, those who are HIV positive and publicly own up to it; young women pregnant out of wedlock, the disabled or physically challenged. Some are shunned and scorned for their cultural practices, for instance the uncircumcised in cultures that circumcise. Stigma brings with it devastating mental, social, spiritual, and economic consequences, and suffering for the person who is stigmatized.

We Listen to the Word of God

DETAILS OF THE TEXT

➤ In our text we get a glimpse of a stigmatized condition and the suffering that it engenders. It was generally believed among the Jews and other cultures, that suffering was a curse from God, especially when it was a seemingly righteous person who was suffering. Read chapters 1 and 2 as a background. Ask the congregation to share similar incidents that they have witnessed. It might be those who have been disfigured by fire or road accident.

➤ From chapter 1, we know that Job has the reputation of being a careful and righteous person. Even after his domestic disaster, Job remains steadfast in his faith. However, in this chapter, we see a devastated Job who is depressed, mournful and suffering from a death wish. His changed situation has become odious to him and a stigma. Life has become for him vanity of vanities.

➤ In verses 1-10, Job curses the day he was born and wants it to perish from his historical memory. Birthdays are celebrated, but Job curses his birthday and finds no meaning in it. What are the things that he says should happen to that day?

➤ In verses 11-19, Job states some reasons why his birthday should be cursed. It ushered him in a world of trouble, while in death all are at rest without any social distinctions. See verses 14,17,18 and 19.

➤ In verses 20-26, Job states his existential predicament. He questions why life should be given to the miserable and to the bitter. Having lost interest in life, such people do not die quickly in a natural way. He celebrates death instead of life. He feels hedged by God on all sides. That which he dreaded most is what came to him. So that he is restless, and knows no peace and quietness.

We Apply the Word of God to Ourselves and the Congregation

WHAT CAN WE LEARN?
- We live in a universe of contending powerful forces in which we are often caught up. We must find a sense of direction and purpose. Currently we are caught up in the scourge of HIV/AIDS. There many lonely sufferers and their families who are devastated mentally, spiritually and economically by it.
- While there is a place for silence in one's suffering, there is also need to speak out as honestly as possible about what one is feeling and thinking, even if it means questioning the purpose of one's existence.
- Those who are well should provide a listening ear to those who are suffering, and empathize with them.
- We do not always understand the reason for human suffering.

WHAT CAN WE CONFESS?
- We condemn people living with HIV/AIDS (PLWHAs) out of ignorance. We do not always seek to understand their circumstances and to hear their story.
- We are quick to speak and provide solutions without listening.
- We associate illness and misfortune with sin and God's punishment.

WHAT CAN WE BE THANKFUL FOR?
- That our birth was not an accident and that even if we walk in the path of the shadow of death, the LORD is still our shepherd. (see Psalm 23)
- That God hears and answers prayer.
- That death is not the answer, but rather the answer is victory over death in Christ.

WHAT CAN WE PRAY FOR?
- Those who because of stigma, are suffering from a death-wish;
- Those who are actually suicidal;
- Caregivers for the HIV/AIDS sufferers;
- The orphans and grandparents;
- Grieving parents who have lost their children.

WHAT CAN WE FEEL?
- Ask the congregation to say what feelings this speech by Job evokes.

WHAT CAN WE BE?
- More understanding, more compassionate, more caring and sensitive to those who are suffering from HIV/AIDS.

WHAT CAN WE DO?
- Ask them how they feel and whether they have any fears. Reassure them that, "The present suffering is not worth comparing with the glory that will be revealed in us." (Romans 8:19)
- Assure them that God loves them and that God is not punishing them.
- Start support groups for PLWHA's, widows, orphans and grieving parents.

126

We Apply the Word of God to the Congregation and Society

The Bible makes it very clear that no one is righteous. We are all sinners needing the grace and forgiveness of God. We are all sick. Sin is the fundamental human deformity and predicament. Because of this, there is no moral ground for stigmatizing and discriminating against anyone. Read Romans 8:28 and 31-39.

Song
Like Jairus (Nga ndi Yayiro, Sumu Za Ukhristu No. 281)

As Jairus of old, I beseech you,
With me in haste to come to my home,
There is sickness beyond cure,
Please come quickly to assist me.

Chorus:

Jesus my Saviour, Lo, I beseech you, today
Come to my rescue, Come to my rescue today.

Death and great suffering all confront me,
They are around me, and within me,
And that's why I often forget you,
I beseech you, come and help me.

The day will come when you will call me,
Call me to heaven, your eternal home,
But this moment, it's me calling,
Please come with me and assist me.

(Rev. Charles Chidongo Chinula - Malawi)

Prayer

Giver and sustainer of life,
Thank you that you know,
And understand when we suffer.
You have even taken our infirmities upon yourself;
And with your wounds we are healed.
Grant us faith and courage
When we are overwhelmed.
In the face of great suffering such
As HIV/AIDS, cancer, malaria and traumas of war,
Remove from us a sense of hopelessness,
When life's meaning disappears
Behind the cloud of suffering,
May we focus our attention upon Christ,
Who suffered and yet conquered. Amen

Suggested Objects/symbols/ideas: Blanket, bed-sheet, wheelchair, bed, medicine bottle, sackcloth, sign-post inscribed "UNCLEAN"   By Augustine C. Musopule

STIGMA: NEITHER THIS MAN NOR HIS PARENTS SINNED
Sermon Text: John 9:1-4

Introduction

One of the factors that make the spread of HIV/ AIDS difficult to contain, is the issue of stigma. Many people attach sin to the HIV positive status. Most people who live with HIV do not have the courage to come out in the open, and declare their status for fear of discrimination. There are stories of people who have been rejected by their parents, relatives and friends, simply because they admitted that they were HIV positive. Some have been killed.

Churches in Africa have not helped the situation because they have led the way in the moral persecution of people living with HIV/AIDS. They have accused them of promiscuity, being sinners and many other names. As a result, many people living with HIV/AIDS would rather suffer, or even die alone, rather than go and disclose their situation to a pastor or church people. This is all because the Church has opted for a message of retribution instead of the gospel of love, forgiveness and compassion.

We Listen to the Word of God

DETAILS OF THE TEXT
  > The disciples asked the question: 'Who has sinned, this man or his parents?' This question is typical throughout all generations. People who are victims of circumstances, are often victimized further by being accused of sin.

  > Jesus declares, 'neither,' thereby releasing the man and his family from the clutches of societal condemnation.

We Apply the Word of God to Ourselves and the Congregation

As was the case in Jewish religion/culture, many believe disease, in this case HIV/AIDS, is punishment for sins committed by the person or their family. But Jesus' answer to those who come asking, 'Who has sinned, this man or his parents?' is most liberating.

WHAT CAN WE LEARN?
People suffer from AIDS, poverty, disabilities or whatever condition, not because they have sinned. We who do not have these conditions are not more righteous or better than those who suffer from them. Suffering is a mystery that cannot be explained away by using our prejudice against the sufferer. The stigma against people living with HIV/AIDS is unloving and most un-Christian.

The Disciples who asked Jesus about the sin of the man with the disability, were victims of their own ignorance, prejudice and fear of the unknown. They gave a simplistic answer to the problem at hand. Likewise, many of us distort the truth and tell ourselves that HIV/AIDS is a result of God's punishment upon those with the virus. The result of this is that we isolate ourselves from those who live with the virus, and drive them underground. What we can learn from the response of Jesus, is that we should see the HIV/AIDS context as an opportunity to show God's love and care, instead of stigmatization and discriminating against the infected.

WHAT CAN WE CONFESS?
- We have driven away people from the Church and from God, by our 'Holier than thou' attitude;
- We have failed to make our churches loving and welcoming communities where all are embraced, irrespective of their conditions;
- We have not understood the gospel of Jesus Christ which says, 'Love your neighbor', 'Take care of these little ones of mine';
- Up to now, our churches remain unfriendly to people living with HIV/AIDS.

WHAT CAN WE THANKFUL FOR?
- People who are living with HIV/AIDS, regardless of the persecution they receive from the Church and other people;
- The Spirit's invitation to the Church to repent and to mend its ways;
- Coping centers which provide support to people living with HIV/AIDS.

WHAT CAN WE PRAY FOR?
Let us pray:
- Creator God we offer our prayer for people living with AIDS;
- Teach us to listen and to honor their pain and emotions;
- Forgive us for the times when we have held them hostage, by accusing them of being immoral and not worthy of mercy;
- We pray that you may help us to learn from the experience.

Song

Amazing graze, how sweet the sound,
That saved a wretch like me.
I once was lost, but now I'm found,
Was blind, but now I see.

That was grace that taught my heart to fear,
And grace my fear relieved.
How precious did that grace appear,
The hour I first believed.
Through many dangers, toils and snares,
I have already come,
Gods' grace has brought me safe thus far,
And he will lead me home.

When we've been there then thousand years,
Bright shinning as the sun.
We've no less days to sing God's praise,
Than when we first begun.

(© John Newton)

Suggested idea: Have members of the congregation do a role-play. This could be a woman who is living with AIDS coming into church to beg for some food. She is emaciated, hungry and a little insane because the virus has infected her brain. As she gets into church, people move away from her and choose to sit somewhere else. She is a little disruptive as she begs during the service. Then two strong men come and throw her out.

By Moiseraele P. Dibeela

GENDERED STIGMA
Sermon Text: Leviticus 12:1-8 and 15:19-24

Menstruation, which begins at puberty and ends with menopause, is a woman's monthly discharge of blood and tissue that has built up during the previous month in the womb. This tissue lines the womb in preparation for the growth of a baby in case of conception, but is discharged when conception has not taken place. This discharge gives opportunity for the development of a new lining and the possibility of pregnancy in the coming month. This is a very powerful experience that only women go through, yet Malawian traditions socially exclude women going through such an experience from routine, until she is considered "normal" again afterwards. The same exclusion happens with post-child birth discharges. She is basically excluded at two levels of her community life: daily routine and worship.

In Leviticus we find a similar view. These culturally gendered perspectives stigmatize women's bodies. They equate women's bodies with uncleanness, hence disease. In HIV/AIDS, this means that women are often the focus of study and the monitoring of the virus. They are more likely to be tested and to know their status than men. This, however, lands many women in trouble. Wives and girlfriends are blamed for bringing the disease home, and sometime they are thrown out, or even killed. At the death of their spouses, even when it was an overt HIV/AIDS case, women still get blamed for witchcraft, and are thrown out of their houses and dispossessed. Stigma breeds violence and isolation. HIV/AIDS certainly has a gendered face, for women's bodies have always been regarded as unclean.

We Listen to the Word of God

Menstruation is a biological process, and is linked to the gift of creating life and is something only women can do. It should be looked at as a gift from God who is sole creator, but who has chosen to share this sacred experience with women. The story of Mary's involvement in the process of God becoming human (incarnation), brings this reality clearly out (Luke 1:26-38). So this is an experience related with fertility, femininity and the joy of bearing children; and is defined as "manner of women", a term free from sinister connotations. It is the joy of womanhood and it is a blessing, not a curse!

DETAILS OF THE TEXT

Leviticus I5:19-24 is an 'ethical' account of how a menstruating woman was supposed to behave according to the Jewish law. According to Mary Douglas, "Proscriptive 'laws' concerning menstruating women (*nidda*), women after childbirth and women with irregular blood issue (*zaba*) are included among the laws of purity and impurity in the book of Leviticus." Nidda as euphemism for "menstruant" might be derived either from the Hebrew root *ndh* (set apart, cast out, banned, separate) or *ndd* (move away), both of which seem to describe the social position of a bleeding woman in regard to her family and society. Such laws have no hygienic connotations, but can be used to: 1) assert male superiority and female inferiority; 2) assert separation of gender roles (Douglas 1966).

In Leviticus 12:1-8 the rituals of cleansing differ depending on the gender of the child born. After the birth of a boy child, the woman is considered unclean for the first seven days like *nidda*, and the next 23 days considered unclean in regard to temple and sacred things only. After the birth of a girl child, however, the woman is considered unclean the first 14 days, and the next 66 days she is unclean in regard to the temple and sacred things. While in the Greek codes the stipulations seem to be characterized by gender asymmetry, the language of exclusion is more stringent towards women and women seem to be seen as a source of pollution.

According to the priestly code, menstrual blood like blood after birth has negative associations. It is considered a major source of defilement. A woman who was menstruating was also described as "ill" and "unwell" (*dawa*). Sex with a menstruating woman, therefore, was considered contaminating, just like illicit sex was. Sex with a menstruating woman as a result of human free choice was considered as an incurable impurity. Within this priestly code, impurity and sanctity (holiness) are interrelated (Leviticus 11:43-44). Sin and guilt offerings are required both from a person who has committed a sin, and from those rendered unclean.

We Apply the Word of God to Ourselves

WHAT CAN WE LEARN?
- Women's bodies are discriminated in many cultures.

WHAT CAN WE CONFESS?
- Our inferiority complexes that have led us to discriminate others whose power scare us.
- Contributing to an environment that makes those whom we discriminate against, live below what God has ordained for them.
- Paralyzing your presence in our communities because of our judgmental attitudes; our gender based stigma in the context of HIV/AIDS.

WHAT CAN WE BE THANKFUL FOR?
- We are your image with dignity, whether women or men;
- Our bodies are your sanctuary, whether in menses or not.

WHAT CAN WE PRAY FOR?
- That God opens our eyes to see God's face in women, even those who are living with AIDS.
- The Holy Spirit to fill us with love, peace, joy, patience, kindness, goodness, faithfulness, humility and self control, so as to be able to minister these banners of service to those around us, despite their experiences.

WHAT CAN WE FEEL?
- Anger at such biases;
- Frustration at the fact that some women have allowed such biases to define them.

WHAT SHOULD WE BE?
- A healing community.

WHAT CAN WE DO?
- Resist such biases through preaching and teachings.
- Affirm women's sexuality and the importance and sacredness of their bodies.

We Apply the Word of God to the Congregation and Society

The community, through both Christian sexuality education institutions and traditional ones, should help girls appreciate their bodies along with the biological processes involved, as God's gift. Menstruation taboos that encourage stigma, like a woman in menses and not putting salt in foods that require salt, should be rid of, while those that ensure safety of the man as well as the woman, should be encouraged to be observed by both (woman in menses, as well as a man with a discharge).

Song
Just as I am, without one plea

Just as I am without one plea,
But that Thy blood was shed for me,
And that Thou bidd'st me come to Thee,
O Lamb of God I come, I come.

Just as I am, though tossed about,
With many a conflict, many a doubt,
Fighting's, fears within, without,
O Lamb of God I come, I come.

Just as I am-poor, wretched, blind-
Sight, riches, healing of the mind,
Yea, all I need, in Thee to find,
O Lamb of God I come, I come.

Just as I am-Thou wilt receive,
Wilt welcome, pardon, cleanse, relieve,

Because Thy promise I believe,
O Lamb of God I come, I come.

Just as I am-Thy love unknown,
Has broken every barrier down;
Now to be Thine, yes, Thine alone,
O Lamb of God I come, I come.

Prayer

A leader asks the people participating in this worship to pray for each and every part of their bodies, while touching each part as they silently pray for it. This action helps emphasize the fact that each part of our body is a member of the temple of the Living God, so we can commit it to our God who created it. In conclusion, after giving enough time to pray for each part of the body, the leader can start the prayer that was taught by Jesus. Each member can be asked to pray in his or her own language.

Suggested Objects: Strings of red beads, white beads, etc.

By Fulata L. Moyo

9. Sexuality

THE GIFTS OF SEXUALITY: "LET HIM KISS ME..."
Sermon Text: Songs of Songs: 1:1-7

Opening Prayer

My dear people,
Let us love one another,
Since love comes from God,
And everyone who loves
Is begotten of God and knows God,
Anyone who fails to love,
Can never have known God. (I John 4:7-11)

Song
An appropriate song of love may be sung.

Introduction

The HIV/AIDS pandemic is forcing us to think and talk about sexuality more often and more openly than before. Sexuality is no longer just a private matter for an individual to ponder in isolation, because one of the consequences of human sexual expression today is HIV/AIDS. However, by sexuality, we must understand more than sex or lovemaking. Sexuality includes reference to all notions, words, gestures and organs considered sexual. In a world where sexuality has been either pushed into the private sphere, or perverted into obscenity, it is important for the church to speak and to comment on what sexuality is or aught to be about. For too long the church has shied away from speaking about sexuality. The devastation of the HIV/AIDS epidemic is such that we can no longer keep silent. Equally important is the question of romantic love - a special and unique gift that God has bestowed upon us. One of the effects of the HIV/AIDS epidemic has been to make people fearful of falling in love, and distrusting of love. As a result, there has been growing lovelessness in our societies. Because of concern about the spread of HIV/AIDS, much focus has been on sex and condoms, and less on love. We believe that love is as important, if not more. It could be that in reaction to the HIV/AIDS epidemic, we are spending too much time and energy teaching (safer) sex, and less time on love. Should the former not be a servant the latter? The church cannot look on as sexuality and love as perverted, for narrow hedonistic aims.

We Listen to the Word of God

Read from Song of Songs 1:1-7
DETAILS OF THE TEXT
This passage contains a shameless and explicit declaration of love by a woman for a man. It is not a passage we often hear or read at church. But why not? Romantic love is something created by God and it aught to be celebrated. What is more, if this passage is anything to go by, both men and women have a right to speak shamelessly and explicitly about their feelings of love. In this passage we meet a woman who is not afraid to express herself as a sexual being, and to see her lover as a sexual being as well. Nor does she hide her desire for the man whom she loves.

We Apply the Word of God to Ourselves

WHAT CAN WE LEARN?
- That sexuality and love are gifts from God which aught to be celebrated;
- That sexuality is beautiful;
- That it is appropriate to speak honestly and openly about love and sexuality;
- That both men and women are free to express themselves on love and sexuality.

WHAT DO WE HAVE TO CONFESS?
- That the church has had a phobia for talking about sexuality and love;
- That we have looked on as others in society as having distorted love and sexuality;
- That in response to the HIV/AIDS epidemic, we might have spent more effort talking about sex but not enough effort on love and sexuality.

WHAT CAN WE BE THANKFUL FOR?
- That God created us as sexual beings and that is part and parcel of having been created in the image of God;
- For the gift of love, even in the times of HIV/AIDS.

WHAT CAN WE PRAY FOR?
- We pray for the church to become bolder in its engagement with matters of sexuality and love;
- We pray for a balance between talk about (safer) sex and talk about romantic love, especially when talking to young people.

We Apply the Word of God to the Congregation

WHAT CAN WE FEEL?
- We feel relieved that there are sections of the Bible that speak openly about sexuality and love, indicating that it is appropriate for us to do the same.

WHAT CAN WE BE?
- We must accept ourselves as sexual beings who can and should fall in love;

WHAT CAN WE DO?
- We can encourage Christians and theirs churches to speak more freely about matters of love and sexuality.

Conclusion: A Word to Society

If we are to succeed in our campaigns against HIV/AIDS, we shall have to deal with the philosophical and cultural barriers that prevent open and honest talk about sexuality and love in the church. Young people cannot be handed over to television and cinema to be taught about sexuality and love. The Bible is very explicit about matters of love and sexuality, we aught to be and do the same.

Prayer of Commitment
Lord makes us brave to speak about sexuality and love in the church. We ask that you to transform your church to be able to shed centuries of shyness about sex, to openly confront issues of sexuality. Above all, we ask that the church become an important institution for love education. All this we ask in the name of Jesus Christ our Lord. Amen

Song
An appropriate love song may be sung

Symbols/objects/ideas and commitments: Roses, candles and drawings of hearts, play a love song, roses, or any appropriate symbols of love.

By Tinyiko S. Maluleke

SEXUALITY: "I AM MY BELOVED'S"
Sermon Text: Song of Songs 7:1-13

Introduction

Sexuality explores the sexual dimension of human life. God created human beings with powerful sexual feelings, although these can be controlled. However, in the historical development of Christianity, a negative attitude towards sexuality has tended to dominate. As a consequence, the link between sexuality and spirituality has been severed. Most African cultures, however, used rites of passage to impart lessons on sexuality to young people. The demonisation of sex, the portrayal of women as temptresses, and negative attitudes towards the human body are significant themes in developing appropriate responses.

It is not surprising that Song of Songs has been "decanonised" by default. Due to a rather conservative and puritanical approach to human sexuality, this sacred text has continued to play a minimal role in the life of the church. It challenges Christians to talk about sexuality realistically and to acknowledge its potency. Issues relating to condom use, pornography, child sexual abuse and others should be openly discussed as we search for godly ways of expressing our sexuality, especially in the HIV/AIDS context.

We Listen to the Word of God

The passage serves to celebrate a woman's body and its power to attract. It acknowledges the reality and force of sexual attraction, recognizing it is a divine creation. It also highlights the centrality of sexuality in a loving relationship. The text identifies female erogenous zones and encourages couples to discover each other. This appreciation of one's partner curtails behavior that increases exposure to HIV/AIDS.

We Apply the Word of God to Ourselves

WHAT CAN WE LEARN?
- Sexuality is God's gift to humanity;
- Couples need to appreciate each other;
- Christians need to break the silence concerning sexuality, particularly in the era of HIV/AIDS.

WHAT DO WE HAVE TO CONFESS?
- Negative attitudes towards sexuality, including the tabooing of any open discussion;
- That many men and women have exposed their partners to HIV/AIDS;
- That celebration of the female body has resulted in pornography;
- That the aspect of love has been removed from most sexual encounters;
- Failing to be romantic in marriage, leading to unfaithfulness;
- Abusing the sexual instinct and increasing the spread of HIV/AIDS;
- The commercialization of women's bodies, leading to rape.

WHAT CAN WE BE THANKFUL FOR?
- God created sexual feelings within us;
- The many individuals who remain faithful;
- That we all have full control over our sexual desires.

WHAT CAN WE PRAY FOR?
- That we may recognize the potency of sexuality in our lives and act responsibly. We should pray for more information and debate concerning this important aspect of our lives. We also ask for the power to abstain and to be faithful, but most importantly, to find ways that will make us enjoy our relationship with our partners.

We Apply the Word of God to the Congregation

Highlight the importance of opening debate on sexuality. With the congregation, identify factors that have led to the demonisation of sexuality. It is also important to illustrate the stigma that emerges from associating HIV/AIDS exclusively with sexuality.

Conclusion: A Word on Society

Mutually faithful loving relationships go a long way in checking the spread of HIV/AIDS. Society needs to recover positive attitudes on sexuality, without succumbing to promiscuity and commercialisation of sex. In addition, there is need for strategies to counter female sexual abuse, stigma, and uncreative approaches to issues of sexuality.

Song

"Malaika" By Mariam Makeba
Or any popular love song.

Prayer

Holy and loving God,
From whose expert hand we proceed,
We thank you for the gift of sexuality.
We praise you for your mighty works.
Guide us that we may appreciate our bodies,
That we may express our sexuality in a responsible way.
Lead us to accept that we are temples of the Holy Spirit.
Forgive us when we minimize your creation.
Teach us to avoid abusing the power of sexual attraction.
Give us courage to denounce all systems that commercialize human bodies.
By your Spirit, enable us to cherish our sexuality
Through Jesus Christ we pray. Amen

Suggested Objects/symbols/ideas: Roses (love); perfume; carving of an embracing couple, beads, indigenous calabash of love, you may read any popular poem on human love and attraction, or any object that symbolizes love in your community.   By Ezra Chitando

SEXUALITY: "I WOULD KISS YOU..."
Sermon Text: Song of Songs 8:1-10

Introduction

Although the book of Song and Songs is very positive about human sexuality, many religious leaders, institutions, and church groups are extremely uncomfortable with issues related to sex, sexuality and sexual health, all of which are closely linked to the HIV/AIDS epidemic in Africa. Talking about sex and sexuality in church is very difficult owing to the historic silence and outright condemnation of these issues by church fathers. Also, African tradition does not seem to be encouraging of open and free discussion of such issues. The fact that HIV/AIDS was first found among homosexuals did not help matters, for HIV/AIDS came to be seen as a judgment from God against sexual immorality. In other instances, church leaders simply lack accurate information to inform their teachings and sermons. Traditional ways of preparing young people in the area of sex, sexuality and sexual health have been challenged by rapid urbanization, cultural change, poverty in the cash economy, selfishness, excessive ambition, greed, war, commercialization of sex, stigma and discrimination based on gender, age and social status.

Many of our sermons therefore do not address the issue of sexuality, and when they do, they are based on suspicion, fear and church tradition, rather than reason, conviction and revelation. With HIV/AIDS related funerals occurring daily, AIDS orphans increasing and our family structures slowly but steadily collapsing, the mission of breaking the silence and discomfort surrounding issues of sexuality cannot be postponed any further.

We Listen to the Word of God

Choose someone to read the Songs of Songs 8:1-10

DETAILS OF THE TEXT
The whole text celebrates the intimate and constant attraction to married or betrothed partners.
Verses 1- 7:
➤ These are strong explanations of love and sexual feelings between rightful partners. The expressions do not provoke feeling of guilt, fear or shame. Nor do they cause the bride and bridegroom to hide their "love talk," or their practical consummation of it. By contrast, wrongful sexual advances and unions are in one way or the other always accompanied by the feelings of guilt, shame, remorse, self hate and emptiness. He/she has let down themselves, their parents, children, friends, guardians, teachers, rightful spouses and God, whether the sexual advances and unions lead to HIV/AIDS or not. Consequently, such sexual unions are usually accompanied by hiding in the "bush"; under the desks in the classroom or office, in the lodge, in friends and neighbors' homes, and in dark corners of gardens or disco halls.

Verse 8-10:

➤ Explain the important fact that girls and boys are expected to preserve their virginity until their wedding day – this is the use of the words "wall" and "door" in Verse 9 and Verse 10. If she is a wall (virgin) we will build upon her a battlement of silver (but if she is a door; has lost her virginity, we will enclose her in brands of cedar). Virginity, however, is also expected from boys.

Verse 10:

➤ The bride takes pride in her virginity and the consequent happiness the bridegroom felt. "I was a wall, and my breasts were like towers, then I was in his eyes as one who brings peace."

We Apply the Word of God to Ourselves

WHAT CAN WE LEARN?

- The creation of human kind in two sexes (man and woman) was not accidental, or an after thought, but God's great intention and purpose.
- Sexual unions (in marriage) were intended by God to offer psychological, physical, emotional and social satisfaction, and spiritual lessons apart from increasing the human race.
- Premarital sexual intercourse (whether it leads to marriage or not) was viewed with great dismay throughout Bible times among God fearing people.
- Premarital sexual relations, adultary and the sex industry are still wrong today, as they were in the Bible times. They are all wrong, even if one avoids being caught, contracting STD's, HIV/AIDS or unwanted pregnancies.

WHAT DO WE CONFESS?

- We have not upheld the positive view of sexuality portrayed by the Bible.
- We have not properly explained the beauty and mystery of sex, sexuality and healthy relationships.
- We have dwelt mostly on the negative aspects of sex and sexuality.
- We have separated issues of "love" from issues of "sex."
- We have demonized sex and sexuality.

WHAT CAN WE BE THANKFUL FOR?

- That God created men and women for each other;
- That the Song of Songs is recorded for us in the Bible;
- That we have leaders, parents and individuals who have tried to put issues of sexuality into their rightful context.

WHAT CAN WE PRAY FOR?

- That God gives us wisdom to teach about what is right and what is safe about sex, sexual acts and relationships in the light of HIV/AIDS.

We Apply the Word of God to the Congregation and the World

WE LOOK AT THE SITUATION OF OUR LISTENERS
- Many are too shy about communicating issues on sex, sexuality and sexual health;
- Many do not differentiate between right and safe celebrations of our sexuality;
- Many are not trained in communicating accurate facts and skills to their children as demanded by Proverbs 22:6.

WE PREACH GOD'S LAW
- Proverbs 22:6 says, "Train the child in the way they should go and even when they grow old; they will never depart from it". So, "If we are silent about sexual issues, young people are neglected and our offspring become as wild beasts, it will be in the fault of our silence and we shall have to render full account of it" (Luther, vol. 46. and The Christian in society, Part 3 page 218).
- If the Christian family cannot give answers to teenagers, the family will lose them to someone who can. If the church is silent, the church will loose them as well.
- Do not criticize God's work or call evil that which God has called well (Genesis 2:18).

WE PREACH GOD'S LAW
- In Luke 2:52 Jesus grows in wisdom, physical, social and spiritual health. Indeed the vigor and strength of a Christian community depends upon the health of its children, youths, couples and elders.
- Song of Songs reminds us that human sexuality is one of the most beautiful aspects of all the divine plans for humanity.
- Ignorance, misconceptions and inappropriate views about sex, sexuality and sexual health need to be at the core of concerns for Christians and their leaders.

Song
Choose any appropriate song.

Prayer
Dear God, we thank you the creator. You made us the temple of your Spirit. You made us sexual beings. Help us to be responsible and express our sexuality openly. Help us to enjoy our sexuality in rightful relationships. Help us to teach our children about responsible sexuality. Help us fight HIV/AIDS. In Jesus name, we pray. Amen

Suggested Ideas/symbols: Heart shapes, roses, beads, flowers, love songs, etc.

By Canon Gideon Byamugisha

10. Reconciliation

Sermon Text: Luke 15:11-32

Prayer

This is the great new problem of humankind. We have inherited a large house, a great "world house" in which we have to live together - black and white, Easterner and Westerner, Gentile and Jew, Catholic and Protestant, Moslem and Hindu - a family unduly separated by ideas, cultures and interests, who, because we can never again live apart, must learn somehow, to live with each other in peace" (Martin Luther King Jr., cited in *Coming Together/Coming Apart. Religion, Community and Modernity,* 1997. Bounds, Elizabeth M. New York: Routledge, p.1).

Lord, we recognize that we live in a polarized world. It is a world divided between white and black, men and women, children and adults, rich and poor, HIV positive and HIV negative people - a world of national and ethnic divisions. We pray for an end to these divisions, which are tearing communities apart. We pray especially for reconciliation between humans and the rest of creation. We ask for wisdom and courage from you Lord, so we may acknowledge the reality of these divisions, confront their bases and seek to overcome them.

Song

An appropriate song on the theme of reconciliation may be sung.

Introduction

One of the effects of HIV/AIDS is to further complicate the division and alienation that is already in society. A whole new set of 'untouchables' has been added the category which already includes blacks, women, the poor, etc. The new group of alienated people are those with HIV/AIDS. What is worse, the suspicion is enough to trigger discrimination. Therefore, HIV/AIDS has thrown communities into further division. Not only do rich countries - whose HIV/AIDS rates are declining and under control - treat the incidence of HIV/AIDS in other countries as if it was not a priority, some of them are directly or indirectly adding HIV/AIDS status as an immigration requirement for people coming from poor countries. There are recorded incidents of people who have been disowned by friends and kin after disclosing their HIV status. But people do not have to be infected with the virus for its devastating effects to be felt. The possibility and fear of HIV/AIDS infection alone, has ensured that people live in suspicion of one another and levels of trust have reached an all time low. There are low levels of trust and high levels of alienation in many communities. Reconciliation is therefore emerging as an important message for the Christian church to proclaim.

We Listen to the Word of God

We read Luke 15: 11-32.
DETAILS OF THE TEXT
One of the reasons this story is so popular and unforgettable, is that it tells a very realistic human story. It was sparked off by a demand from the younger son to cut ties with his father. So he sets off with his inheritance. Modern commentators may see the younger son's push for independence as positive. They may chastise the older son for his continuing dependency on the father. They will most probably praise the father for letting go - something that is often difficult for parents. (One wonders about the mother and other siblings - have they been edited out of the parable because they are women? It would have been interesting to know their views and roles in the development of this story.) Indeed, even though the younger son's time of independence is later shown to have failed dismally, some may still argue that he came back wiser than he would have, had he not ventured out into the unknown. This line of interpretation displays the younger son and the father in good light, and the older son in very bad light. We miss a crucial point in the story, if all we do is to try and sort out the good son from the bad son. Nor is it helpful to proceed by generating a list of good and bad points of each of the three characters.

An important and basic point in the story is that three people who lived in community and fellowship, lost that community and fellowship. They became alienated one from the other.

Such was the depth and pain of the alienation, that the ending of the story suggests that it no longer mattered who was right and who was wrong. If we were to modernize this story, the younger son could have come back, not only destitute and hungry, but also HIV positive. Without a well balanced diet for so long, his health may have deteriorated rapidly. The father could have chosen to give his son a lengthy, I-told-you-so lecture. But his skinny frame must have stung his father's eyes, so that he immediately had compassion on him. When alienation and enmity runs deep and its ghastly fruits are there for all to see and touch, it may become necessary to go beyond finger-pointing if we are to achieve reconciliation.

This is precisely what the father does. He goes beyond finger pointing. For him, the community that was once shared between him and his sons is far too important to be sacrificed at the altar of an I-told-you-so, self-righteous ethic. At least three members of the broken family have an opportunity to live in community again. Even if the father is ready to try community again and to be reconciled to his son, the two sons appear unsure and reluctant. The younger son suggests that he be henceforth treated as if he was not a son. An astounding suggestion. How does a son get treated as if he was not a son? The older son suggests that the younger son has lost all rights and privileges of brotherhood - calling him 'this son of yours'. Indications are that since the departure of the younger son, the remaining father and son were never able to live in community themselves; at least not in the manner that they had experienced community before. Hence the return of the younger son becomes an occasion for the older son to voice his reservations - reservations he had probably held ever since that fateful day when his younger brother set off into the unknown.

The return of the younger son has potential to reconcile the lost son to the two who remained at home, but also to restore relations between the father and the older son. In this context, is reconciliation and community possible? The father thinks so. His response is that a son is home.

This of course does not mean that he will not sit the son down for a serious heart to heart discussion. It should not mean that he would pretend that the separation never happened. It should not mean that the father would pretend not to be hurt and not to be angry. But all of these are expressed within a context where sons are regarded as such, and encouraged to restore the brotherhood they share. It is a sad day when sons and daughters are treated as if they were hirelings in their own home - whether this is done as punishment, or as a consequence of stigma and discrimination. Reconciliation is a process, but unless the correct starting points and context are set at the beginning, it is likely to remain forever illusive.

We Apply the Word of God and to Ourselves

WHAT CAN WE LEARN?
- We learn that alienation is painful and can go very deep.
- That it is not acceptable for daughters and sons to live as if they were slaves in their own households. Could it be that because of stigma, HIV positive daughters and sons are being treated as if they were slaves and hirelings?
- That it is necessary to go beyond finger pointing if reconciliation is to be initiated. HIV positive people deserve to be reconciled to their spouses, children, extended families, communities and churches.
- Although reconciliation is a process, it is important to create the right context and employ the correct starting points in initiating it. If your son or daughter contract HIV/AIDS, that they are your children is a non-negotiable starting point. They are bearers of the image of God, even as they lie emaciated in hospital beds.

WHAT DO WE HAVE TO CONFESS?
- We confess that we have often failed to grasp the depth and pain of alienation that HIV/AIDS unleashes on families and in communities.
- We confess that we have often gone no further than finger pointing - even in our sermons.
- We confess that we have to strive to ensure that the appropriate context and starting points are in place in order for the reconciliation process to be authentic.
- We confess that some of our churches have ignored times that HIV positive people are treated as 'hirelings' by governments and communities. What is worse is that they have even sometimes been treated as such inside the church.

WHAT CAN WE BE THANKFUL FOR?
- We can be thankful that public opinion is slowly changing about the HIV/AIDS epidemic and as a result, more and more people are willing to fight stigma.
- We can be thankful that some HIV positive people find support from their families, communities and churches.
- More and more governments are taking HIV treatment and prevention very seriously.
- For the millions of health workers and other volunteers who work with HIV positive people and AIDS sufferers.

WHAT CAN WE PRAY FOR?
- For increased awareness of the devastating effect of HIV/AIDS on community, and the alienation that it causes.

- For an increased understanding of the way the virus spreads and the way in which its effects may be postponed.
- For more trust and more hope in communities devastated by the HIV/AIDS pandemic.

We Apply the Word of God to the Congregation

WHAT CAN WE FEEL?
- We should feel inspired to combat HIV/AIDS at the level where it spreads distrust, hopelessness and alienation.
- We should feel concerned that HIV/AIDS tears communities and families apart at so many different levels.

WHAT CAN WE BE?
- We can be brave and bold in the knowledge that the alienating effects of HIV/AIDS can be reversed.

WHAT CAN WE DO?
- We can engage in trust building activities with infected and affected people.

Conclusion: A Word to Society

HIV/AIDS attacks communities. It spreads alienation which causes spouses, parents, children and whole communities to be alienated one from each other. The message of reconciliation has therefore become very important in the work of the church in these times. It is the duty of the church to build bridges between people torn apart by HIV/AIDS. For this to happen, it will be necessary for the church to take people beyond finger pointing, but to do so without refraining from facilitating deep communication and discussion between the infected and the affected.

Prayer of Commitment

My head is heavy, my shoulders shrug
Because despite all my eyes have seen,
My head has said, my heart has felt,
I do not believe
That White, Black and Yellow
Cannot talk, walk, eat, kiss and share ...
(From a poem titled: "An Agony" by Joyce Nomafa Sikakane, reproduced in full by De Gruchy, John 1986. *Cry Justice!* London: Collins, p.155-156)

Song
An appropriate song with the reconciliation theme may be sung.

Symbols/objects/ideas and commitments: The cross, shaking hands and pictures of people hugging.

By Tinyiko Maluleke

11. Healing

Suggested Reading Mark 1:40-42 and Luke 7:20-22

Instructions: In preparation, get your choir or worship leaders to practice the song, giving it the most appropriate tune for the theme of the service and the audience. Assign different readers to read different scriptures and lead with prayers. The aim of this service is to heal its participants: bodily, spiritually, mentally, socially, economically, etc. It also seeks to get participants to realize that HIV/AIDS is an epidemic within other social diseases of poverty, gender inequality, violence, human rights violations, national and international injustice—which must also be healed. If you are in a small group, get people to sit in a circle. If you are in a big worship group, let people sit down where they are. The readers can read where they are seated if their voices are sufficiently clear. Close the service by serving the Lord's Supper as part of the healing process.

Call to Worship

"Surely God is my salvation; I will trust and I will not be afraid, for the Lord God is my strength and might; God has become my salvation." (Isaiah 12:2)

Song
Heal our Land
Or any appropriate song.

    Heal our Land, oh Lord (2x)
    Heal our land (3x)

    Bind our wounds oh Lord (2x)
    Bind our wounds (3x)

    Refodise Morena (2x)
    Refodise Morena (3x)

    Re tle Matshidiso Morena (2x)
    Re tshidise Morena (3x)
        (© Musa W. Dube)

Reader 1:   (Mark 1:40-42)
        A leper came to him begging him, and kneeling he said to him, "If you choose, you can make me clean." Moved with pity, Jesus stretched out his hand and touched him, and said to him, I do choose. Be made clean! Immediately the leprosy left him, and he was made clean.

All: He took our infirmities and bore our diseases,
        And by his stripes and bruises we are healed. (Isaiah 53:4-5)

Reader 2:	(Luke 7:20-22)
	They said to him, "John the Baptist has sent us to you to ask, 'Are you the one who is to come, or are we to wait for another?'… He answered them, "Go and tell John what you have seen and heard: the blind receive sight, the lame walk, the lepers are cleansed, the deaf hear, the dead are raised, the poor have good news brought to them."
All:	He took our infirmities and bore our diseases,
	And by his stripes and bruises we are healed. (Isaiah 53:4-5)

Song
Heal our Land

Heal our Land, oh Lord, (2x)
Heal our land. (3x)

Bind our wounds, oh Lord, (2x)
Bind our wounds. (3x)

Prayer of Confession and Healing

We confess that:
We are a church infected and affected by HIV/AIDS.
We are a church suffering from opportunistic infections.
We are a church living with and dying with HIV/AIDS.
We are a church suffering from stigma and discrimination.
Heal us Lord. Bind our wounds.

We bring our hearts to you for healing.
We bring our souls to you for your healing.
We bring our minds to you for your healing.
We bring our broken hearts and families for healing.
Heal us Lord. Bind our wounds and have mercy on us.

Heal us Lord with your resurrection power.
Cause us to rise from fear and hopelessness.
Cause us to rise into your resurrection hope.
Heal us and fill us with your Spirit of power and life.

Song
You may choose another appropriate song.

Prayer for Holistic Healing

Leader 1:	Heal us from bodily pains of HIV/AIDS,
	That depletes our immunity,
	And leaves us open to opportunistic infections.
	Heal us Lord.
All:	*Clap hands twice*
	Heal us Lord. Have mercy on us.
Leader 2:	Heal us from our broken hearts and grief,
	That continues to pain our spirits and minds
	And leave us empty about the meaning of life.
	Heal us Lord.
All:	*Clap hands twice*
	Heal us Lord. Have mercy on us.
Leader 3:	Heal us from psychological pains of HIV/AIDS,
	That engulf us in fear and hopelessness
	And lead us to die before the virus kills us.
	Heals us Lord.
All:	*Clap hands twice*
	Heal us Lord. Have mercy on us.
Leader 4:	Heal us from HIV/AIDS social stigma and discrimination,
	That leads us to uncompassionate acts of isolation,
	And failure to provide quality care and prevention.
	Heal us Lord.
All:	*Clap hands twice*
	Heal us Lord. Have mercy on us.
Leader 5:	Heal us from unhealthy family relations,
	That tolerate unfaithfulness and hurt family,
	And spreads HIV/AIDS to our loved ones.
	Heal us Lord.
All:	*Clap hands twice*
	Heal us Lord. Have mercy on us.
Leader 6:	Heal us from unhealthy gender relations,
	That exposes partners and spouses to HIV/AIDS infection
	And leaves women powerless to protect themselves.
	Heal us Lord.
All:	*Clap hands twice*
	Heal us Lord. Have mercy on us.
Leader 7:	Heal us from poverty that exposes millions to HIV/AIDS.
	Heal us from exploitative social structures,
	That condemn many to poverty and expose them to infection.
	Heal us Lord.
All:	*Clap hands twice*
	Heal us Lord. Have mercy on us.
Leader 8:	Heal us from violence that spreads HIV/AIDS.
	Heals us from ethnic and civil wars.
	Heal us from domestic violence and the rape of children.
	Heal us Lord.

All:	*Clap hands twice*
	Heal us Lord. Have mercy on us.
Leader 9:	Heal us from national corruption,
	That embezzles funds, tramples on human rights,
	And denies quality health services to its citizens.
	Heal us Lord.
All:	*Clap hands twice*
	Heal us Lord. Have mercy on us.
Leader 10:	Heal us from international injustice,
	That sets up exploitative economic policies of trade
	And denies millions access to HIV/AIDS drugs.
	Heal us Lord.
All:	*Clap hands twice*
	Heal us Lord. Have mercy on us.
	Heal us with your resurrection power.
	Cause us to rise from fear and hopelessness.
	Cause us to rise into your resurrection hope.
	Cause us to reclaim our right to life and to quality life.
	Heal us Lord, fill us with the joy of your Spirit.
	And your peace that surpasses all understanding. Amen

Song

Blessed Assurance, Jesus is Mine
Or any appropriate song.

The Lord's Supper is served

The Eucharist is served as part of our healing.

Song

Sizo hamba naye (Thuma Mina, No. 180)

Prayer

The Lord's Prayer
Each in their own language.

Suggested Objects/symbols/ideas: The Lord's supper or sharing the water of life.

By Musa W. Dube

Part 4
Services for Specific Groups

1. Children
Mark 5:21-43 (Musa W. Dube)
Matthew 2:1-13 (Tinyiko S. Maluleke)
Lucas 18:15-17 (Felicidade N. Cherinda)

2. The Boy-child
Gen. 39:1-10 (Augustine C. Musopule)
Proverbs 4:1-23 (Ezra Chitando)

3. The Girl-child
2 Samuel 13 (Isabel Apawo Phiri)
Judges 11:34-40 (Tinyiko S. Maluleke)

4. Youth
Ecclesiastes 1:7-12:8 (Moiseraele P. Dibeela)

5. Parents and Parenthood
I Samuel 2:2-17 (Cheryl Dibeela)
Matthew 15:21-28 (Musa W. Dube)

6. Men and Fatherhood
Genesis 19:1-11 (Tinyiko S. Maluleke)
Mark 9:33-36 (Ezra Chitando

7. Women
Proverbs 31:10-31 (Ezra Chitando)
Ruth 1-2 (Isabel Apawo Phiri)

8. Widows and Widowhood
Luke 18:1-8 (Musa W. Dube)
Ruth 1:1-22 (Felicidade N. Cherinda)

9. Homosexuals
I John 4:7-21(Musa W. Dube)

10. Persons Living With HIV/AIDS
Jeremiah 17:5-10 (Ezra Chitando)

11. Community Leadership
Nehemiah 1-4 (Cheryl Dibeela)

12. HIV/AIDS Workers
Matt. 9:35-38 and John 21: 15-18 (Musa W. Dube)

1. Children

SERVICES FOR/BY/ON CHILDREN
Suggested Passage: Mark 5:21-43

Instructions: Depending on the context and what the preacher wants to achieve, you may wish to run an interactive service between children and adults. In this case, you may begin by highlighting the different situations confronting children by using the provided poetic opening. Get many different children to read a line of the poem—either from where they are sitting or have them come to the front. This will be followed by the adult response, a song and a sermon. The closing will also be an interactive prayer between children and adults/parents. The preacher may decide to use some of the suggested symbols to highlight the situation of children in difficult circumstances, especially the HIV/AIDS context.

Leader: *Ngwana yo osa le leng a swela tharing //* A child who does not cry out (make her/himself heard) can die on their mother's back.

Poetic Opening

Child 1: I am the child in your house, loved and cared for by you.
Child 2: I am the child in your church, known or unknown to you.
Child 3: I am the child in your schools, passing or failing my subjects.
Child 4: I am a street child, standing beside your roads, dirty and eating from the dumping sites.
Child 5: I am the child targeted by media, drugs and commerce, tempted by sugar daddies and mummies with their money.
Child 6: I am a child soldier in the war-torn zones, carrying a gun and killing.
Child 7: I am the child in a poverty stricken home, sold into slavery and sex work.
Child 8: I am a child in my own home, caring for my sick and dying parents.
Child 9: I am an orphan in a child-headed home, caring for my siblings; facing stigma and an uncertain future.
Child 10: I am a child in your house, sexually molested by relatives and strangers, who want to cleanse themselves of HIV/AIDS.
Child 11: I am the sickly child in your midst, born HIV positive from my infected parents.
Child 12: I am the disabled and physically challenged child, forgotten by your institutions and strategic plans.

All Children: We are children of the world.
We are today's citizens.
We are the speaking children, seeking your hearing.
We are children knocking at your door.
Open the door for us in God's household.

Congregational/Adult Response

Leader: All children are a blessing from God;
All: And it takes a village to raise a child.
Leader: All children are special before God;
All: Help us to be a village that raises children.
Leader: All children are called to come unto Christ;
All: For the kingdom of God belongs to them.
Leader: God welcomes all children;
All: Help us to welcome all children in our homes and churches.

Reading of the text: Mark 5:21-43

Introduction

In many societies and cultures, children are powerless. They do not have the right to speak and to be heard, they are dependent upon their guardians and parents for survival, and they often do not have legal rights or representation in the government. While in the past, parents and elders in most African countries were held to be responsible parents, this can no longer be assumed. Many parents are shackled by wars, poverty, labor immigration, displacement and HIV/AIDS and so are not able to play their roles effectively. This has left many children particularly vulnerable to abuse. The HIV/AIDS epidemic has particularly added to the vulnerability of children as powerless members of their societies. Many are orphaned, grieved and left with no parental guidance or provision, hence open to sexual abuse, labor exploitation, uncertain futures, stigma, discrimination, rape and poverty. We now have child-headed homes, where the children's chances of going to school successfully are often very slim. They become school dropouts, they fall to teenage pregnancy, and face a high chance of HIV/AIDS infection.

In the story of Mark 5:21-43 we are confronted by a desperate parent in search for healing for his child. We also realize that Jesus takes seriously the importance of saving children from death. He walks with a desperate parent to see the dying child. He arrives at the bedside of the dead child and calls a little girl from death to life. The story gives us a good example for parenting in the HIV/AIDS era, where children live under the threat of death. It particularly calls for caring fathers and men to protect the girl child from HIV/AIDS death.

We Listen to the Word of God

DETAILS OF THE TEXT
Verse 21-24:
 > These verses provide the setting and details of the story. Jesus is just landing by the sea and he is surrounded by a crowd. It is in this situation that a desperate parent (Jairus) comes to Jesus.

 > It is important to highlight that Jairus is religious leader, a father and a man. He can become a model for both church leaders and fathers to care and to seek for life and health for their children.

➤ Highlight that this child is also a daughter. The girl child tends to be marginalized and neglected, but both Jairus and Jesus care for her life and health.

➤ Underline that Jesus, despite his fame, walks with Jairus, a desperate parent. Jesus could have pronounced the child well without going there, so it is significant that he takes the time to walk with the parent, to see the sick and dying child.

Verses 25-35:
➤ Jesus is delayed in order to meet the needs of a desperate patient—the bleeding woman, who has been sick for twelve years. This delay leads to the death of the little girl.

➤ Highlight that in a society where many are suffering from incurable diseases, attention to children is inevitably divided.

Verses 36-37:
➤ Note Jesus' response: he gives hope to Jairus. Underline that Jesus says, "Do not fear, only believe." That is, he speaks against hopelessness and fear, and insists on hope.

➤ Jesus courageously confronts death and does not allow it to plant fear and hopelessness.

Verse 38-39:
➤ Note the reality of death, attested by mourning, weeping, wailing and commotion. This confirms the message of the messengers. The little girl is dead.

➤ Highlight how Jesus insists on hope: he still refuses to let death plant fear and grief. He insists on life, "The child is not dead," he says. This is stubborn faith and hope.

Verses 40-43:
➤ Note how Jesus accompanies the parents of the child to where the child is lying.

➤ Highlight that he takes the disciples with him—indicating that such a role is expected from his followers, the church.

➤ Note the touch. Jesus touches the girl. Jesus is not deterred by cultural beliefs that sometimes equate dead bodies with uncleanness. He breaks cultural barriers.

➤ Note that he calls her back to life, from her sleep of death.

➤ It is important to emphasize her response: she rises and starts walking. This point challenges the children themselves—they need to hear the voice of Christ calling them from death to life.

➤ Jesus commands that she should be given food. This an important point to emphasize, especially since many children die due to hunger and starvation.

➤ In sum, underline that Jesus refuses to let death and hopelessness have the final word. He refuses to let death overcome children. He refuses to let hunger and illness destroy

153

children. He accompanies desperate parents and calls children to life. The church needs to play this role in the HIV/AIDS era.

We Apply the Word of God to Ourselves

WHAT CAN WE LEARN?
- We should not give up searching for the healing of our children;
- We need to walk with desperate parents to their homes;
- We can call our children from death to life;
- Children can learn to appreciate their parents' care;
- Children can learn to hear the voice of Christ that calls them from death to life.

WHAT DO WE HAVE TO CONFESS?
Prayer of confession:
- We confess that we have not always been a good village for children to grow up in;
- We confess that we are not always a child-friendly church in our services;
- In the HIV/AIDS era we have exposed children to sexual violence and rape;
- We confess that orphaned children are abused, exploited and stigmatized;
- We confess that we have not been a parenting church to child-headed homes;
- We confess that we have not fed the orphans or provided for their needs;
- We confess that we have not reached out to the grieved child;
- Help us Lord to welcome children as we welcome the One who sent you.

WHAT CAN WE BE THANKFUL FOR?
- For our children;
- For a God who welcomes children;
- For parents who are struggling to raise and provide for their children;
- For grandmothers who are parenting orphaned children;
- For governments, NGOs and agencies that work for children's wellbeing.

WHAT CAN WE PRAY FOR?
- For a parenting church;
- For churches that are child-friendly in all of their departments;
- For leadership in providing for the needs of orphaned children;
- For governments to provide legal protection for children in the HIV/AIDS era.

We Apply the Word of God to the Congregation

WHAT CAN WE BE?
- A child-friendly and parenting church.

WHAT CAN WE DO?
- Set up child-friendly services in the church;
- Set up day-care centers for orphaned children;
- Set up feeding and counseling services for needy and grieving children, especially orphans;

- Collaborate with NGOs and agencies that work with children's needs;
- Put pressure on our governments to legally protect all children;
- Put pressure on governments to rectify and implement the Convention on Children's rights.

Conclusion: A Word on Society

While most societies, cultures and families are still not used to, or open to, the concepts of children's rights, the wide abuse and exploitation of children underlines the need for children's rights education. In particular, the rubbishing of children, manifested by the rape of young girls by men and male relatives who seek to cleanse themselves of HIV/AIDS, underlines the need to protect the rights of children, particularly the girl child. The Christian church can seek to become a parenting church, a church that calls for fathers to protect their girl children, and a church that insists on calling children from death to life. The church can become advocates for children's rights. Like Jairus, church leaders must take a lead role in protecting children.

While it cannot be assumed that the church subscribes to children rights, the gospel compels Christians to protect children. In particular, Jesus said, "Let the children come to me, and do not hinder them, for the kingdom of God belongs to them" (Mark 10:13-16). He also said, "Whoever welcomes one of these little children in my name, welcomes me and whoever welcomes me, welcomes not me but the one who sent me" (Mark 9:37). These scriptures are sufficient to give the church a theology that protects children in the wider society, especially in this HIV/AIDS era.

Song
The Sun is Rising Upon Africa

You can chant this song in a poetic form, or get some youth to rap it with their own tune, or choose another suitable song.

Lead voice:
The sun is rising upon Africa,
The sun has risen upon Africa,
The sun is blooming upon Africa,
The whole continent is wearing light.

All voices:
Yea, shine my heart, lay my heart, sing my heart, laugh my heart, jump heart
For God liveth. (3x)
Yea, ring my heart, harp, drum, dance, clap, smile, play
For God liveth (3x) God liveth (2x)

Lead voice:
The sun is rising upon Botswana,
The sun has risen upon the skies of Botswana,
The sun is shinning upon the face of Botswana,
The whole nation is wearing light,
For God liveth (2x) God liveth (2x)

All voices:
Yea, shine my child, play my child, laugh my child, jump my child, shout my heart,
For God liveth (3x)
Yea, ring my child, hard, drum, dance, clap, smile, play,
For God liveth (3x) God liveth (2x)

The sun is rising upon my heart,
The sun has risen upon my soul,
The sun is shining upon my my brows,
My whole body is wearing light,
For God liveth (3x) God liveth (2x)

Yea, shine my heart…

(© Musa W. Dube)

Responsive Prayer

Children:
Like the little girl at the point of death,
Many of us are dying in the HIV/AIDS context.
Talitha cum, children let us rise from death.

Parents/All adults:
Like Jairus, we are coming to you Jesus, we are calling you,
We fall before you, we beg you repeatedly.
Come to our homes and save our dying children.
Walk with us in our fear and grief.
Save our children from disease and death.

Children:
God our friend, you understand and you listen to us.
Many of us are dying due to peer pressure.
Many of us are exposed to drugs and alcohol abuse.
Many of us are dying due to early and inappropriate sex.
We are dying because we disregard our parents, guardians and teachers.
Help us to hear your voice calling us to life.

Parents/Adults:
Talitha cum! Children, arise from death, for Jesus is calling you.

Children:
Help us to see you standing by our beds of sickness and death,
Help us to feel your power of life when you touch our hands,
Help us hear your voice when you call us from death to life,
Help us to rise from death to life.

All: ๛
Help us Lord,
Help us to call *Talitha Cum* to all dying children,
We pray and ask this in Jesus name.

Suggested Symbols/objects/ideas: Tell an African folktale about children or proverbs; a poster of a hatching egg; play Sibongile Khumalo's "Little girl when the time comes," from the *Ancient Evenings* album; tell the story of Nkosi, the child HIV/AIDS activist from South Africa; have some children recite Mark 9:37 and Mark 10:14; or use whatever idea and symbols that may be appropriate to your context and audience.

By Musa W. Dube

KEEPING CHILDREN FROM HARM
Sermon Text: Matthew 2:1-13

Opening Prayer/Poem

Soweto sprawls beneath the stars,
While Herod sleeps,
Although they're late, the hours he keeps,
In curfew'd caution,
And, warned in dreams of other roads,
I never told him,
That I found the Infant Christ ...
Black arms enfold Him.
What black? What notion?
The dust had settled, satin-soft,
On dongas, quilted,
Above the little shoe-box house,
The Star had halted. ...

(Extracted from the poem titled, "The Black Madonna" by Maria Mackay OP, published in the journal *Grace and Truth* no. 1, 1993, p.38 and 39.)

Song
An appropriate song on God's love for children and their welfare may be sung.

Introduction

We live in a world where danger encircles children from the day they are born. HIV/AIDS is a case in point, as many children are born HIV positive. In times past, African people were very much awake to the dangers of infection and disease that threatened newly born babies. Consequently they went to great lengths to ensure that the infant was protected. For example, an infant was not allowed out of the house of birth for weeks, if not months, after birth. When eventually the infant came out of the house, there would be ritual and ceremony designed to protect the child further. It is interesting to note that God went to great lengths to ensure that the child Jesus was protected and kept from harm. How much trouble do we take to ensure that our newborns are kept from harm? What are governments in Africa doing to reduce infant mortality rates? What are they doing to prevent mother to child HIV transmission? What are men and women who are sexually active doing to prevent the transmission of HIV/AIDS to newly born babies? How far do we go in protecting children and keeping them from harm? The recent and chilling spate of infant rapes by men who believe this to be a cure for AIDS, has once again highlighted the vulnerability of infant children to HIV/AIDS.

We Listen to the Word of God

We read from Matthew 2:1-13
DETAILS OF THE TEXT
The news of the birth of Jesus the Messiah was not received well by Herod. In fact, the news caught him unawares. It was when the Magi came looking for the child that Herod learned of the birth. He takes immediate action and enlists the services of the Magi to help him trace the whereabouts of the child, in the pretense that he too wished to worship him. Ordinarily the birth of a child should bring joy. But we are told that the birth of this child disturbed Herod and all of Jerusalem. Basically Herod and the inhabitants of Jerusalem saw the child Jesus as a threat to their power and positions. But God did not take chances with the safety of this child. First, God intervenes by visiting the Magi in a dream advising them to return to their country by another route, so as to avoid sharing the information of the child's whereabouts with Herod. Secondly, God intervened more decisively in yet another dream to Joseph saying: "Get up, take the child and its mother, and escape to Egypt. Stay there until I tell you". It is these two decisive and timely interventions, which ensure that the infant Jesus lives to see another day. Had God not intervened decisively, Herod might have succeeded in bring a premature end to Jesus' life.

Furthermore, it is noteworthy that both the Magi and Joseph cooperate when God advises them to change routes and to escape respectively. Are we prepared to change our ways - i.e. to come back by a different route - even if we may have to trod unfamiliar and inconvenient alternative routes for the sake of keeping our children from harm? Would we remove ourselves from familiar territories and move elsewhere for the sake of our children? It seems to me that this is what the HIV/AIDS epidemic demands of us: first that we align ourselves and cooperate with God's vision and love for children, and that we be prepared to try alternative routes from the tried and trusted ones with which we are familiar.

We Apply the Word of God

WHAT CAN WE LEARN?
- That infants are a most vulnerable group;
- From the passage we learn that infants are dependant on parents and adults for protection;
- That God intervened decisively in order to protect the infant Jesus;
- We also note the manner in which the adults in the life of Jesus cooperated with God's vision and love for children;
- The HIV/AIDS pandemic requires extra efforts from parents and adults in protecting children from harm.

WHAT DO WE HAVE TO CONFESS?
- We confess widespread and gross neglect of infant children in our societies;
- We confess the refusal of adults and children to engage in extra and unfamiliar efforts for the sake of keeping infants from harm;
- We confess the widespread and growing abuse of infants;
- We confess that due to adult, parental, societal and governmental neglect many children are needlessly born HIV positive.

WHAT CAN WE BE THANKFUL FOR?
- For the gift of childbirth and of infants.
- For the millions of parents and adults who care enough for infants that they are willing to try routes and territories other than the familiar.
- That God has given us clues as to how we should treat infants during our own times.

WHAT CAN WE PRAY FOR?
- For a world in which infants matter;
- For world in which extra-ordinary measures will be taken in order to keep infants from harm;
- For societies and parents who will intervene and do so courageously in order to save infants;
- For a world in which no infant will be born HIV positive.

We Apply the Word of God to the Congregation

WHAT CAN WE FEEL?
- Sorrow for the horrendous and untold suffering meted out to infant children;
- Ashamed that we do not always do enough to keep children from danger;
- Inspired by the example of parents and adults in Matthew 2 who cooperated with God in order to save the life of the child Jesus.

WHAT CAN WE BE?
- We can become better parents;
- We can become a society that is more caring for children;
- We can become a society in which no child is born HIV positive.

Conclusion: A Word to Society

The HIV/AIDS scourge places an extra challenge on us insofar as protecting children is concerned. HIV/AIDS is not content with mowing down young men and women at their prime. It also attacks newly born babies - ensuring that they do not live long enough to see their teens. HIV/AIDS is the new Herod that seeks to smother and extinguish the promise that infants hold. It is the new 'conspiracy' designed to end the lives of human beings at the infant stage. We must do all in our power to protect this most vulnerable and innocent group of victims of HIV/AIDS. Governments, parents, community organizations, churches and societies at large, should leave no stone unturned in the search for practices that will keep children from this particular danger.

Prayer of Commitment

Lord, we commit ourselves to seeking alternative lifestyle routes that will ensure that innocent infants do not become victims of HIV/AIDS. We commit ourselves to cooperate with God who loves children. Help us, oh Lord to become parents who are worthy and adults who act responsibly towards vulnerable infants. In the name of Christ we pray, Amen

Song

Sing an appropriate song focusing on infants and the role of adults in providing for them.

Symbols/objects/ideas: Cradle, cot.

By Tinyiko S. Maluleke

SERVIÇO PARA CRIANÇAS
Texto Sugerido: Lucas 18:15-17

Introdução

Na cultura africana, as crianças não devem ficar onde os adultos se encontram. Faz-se isso para evitar que se transformem em mentirosas ou incómodas pelo barrulho que podem fazer. O que é negativo é que esse afastamento acaba por afectar as relações entre pais e filhos. As crianças crescem sem nenhuma orientação e acabam aprendendo sobre a vida por pessoas não indicadas. Os pais não rezam com so seus filhos nem os levam à igreja para serem abençoadas. Procedendo dessa maneira, como é que podem receber e ajudar crianças infectadas e afectadas pelo HIV/SIDA? As igrejas tentam integrá-las em muitos programas e preparam-nas para o futuro. Todavia, muitas vezes essa preparação é feita por outras crianças. Isso não seria contestado se antes fossem bem treinadas para o efeito. Como muitas vezes isso não acontece, são poucas as que participam activamente e acabam por abandonar. Jesus critica essa atitude dizendo que os adultos devem deixar as crianças irem ter com Ele, porque é deles o Reino dos Céus. Hoje em dia, as crianças estão em perigo. Crescem sem amor, sem nessecidades básicas, são infectadas, raptadas, violadas, a sua situação é deveras crítica. Precisamos de protegê-las, de conhecer e de aplicar os seus direitos. Precisamos de escutar e seguir o que o texto diz. Uma criança bem instruída e orientada é garantia de vida harmoniosa e de paz.

Vamos Escutar a Palavra de Deus

Leia o texto. Sublinhe com um lápis as palavras mais importantes.

QUE PODEMOS APRENDER?
- Que tal como acontecia com os discípulos, a sociedade não tem acesso aos seus dirigentes porque aqueles que estão perto deles, criam dificuldades. Figuras públicas acabam ficando impopulares.
- Que Jesus não gosta que alguém seja impedido (a) de ir ter com Ele.
- Jesus realça que o Reino de Deus é para toda gente.

QUE PODEMOS CONFESSAR?

- Que muitas vezes não temos interesse pelas crianças, não lhes proporciamos a devida atenção.
- Que as excluímos em muitas actividades nas nossas igrejas.
- Que não ajudamos as nossas crianças a saber escolher o que é bom para elas.
- Que usamos as crianças para resolver os nossos problemas económicos.

Palavra de Deus para a Sociedade

O texto fala de discriminação baseada no género e na idade.Alguns textos da Bíblia relatam acontecimentos em que havendo necessidade de conhecer o número de pessoas presentes, as mulheres e as crianças não são contadas (Ex.Mt 14.21). Mulheres e crianças são tidas como objectos. Fazem parte da propriedade dos homens.Isso é uma discriminação, é uma opressão. A atidude de Jesus ensina-nos que no Reino de Deus, todos tem lugar e são importantes.Jesus quer crianças ao pé de si , porque são muito activas. As crianças fazem muitas perguntas, querem saber tudo.Os adultos calam-se. Como vão conhecer a vontade de Deus? Como vão aprender novas coisas e modificar o mundo? Jesus conclui dizendo que quem não for como uma criança, não vai entrar no Reino de Deus.

CANÇÂO

Escolher uma que fala de crianças

ORAÇÂO

Glória e louvor sejam dados ao nosso Deus.Senhor, tu que és Um Deus que ama, que liberta, que consola, que perdoa. Estamos aqui para pedir a tua orientação. Precisamos que nos ensines a escutar o grito daqueles que choram, daqueles que lutam pela igualdade de direitos, daqueles que se batem por um mundo melhor. Senhor, faça de nós instrumentos da tua paz, hoje e para sempe. Amen.

Objectos: Uma fotografia com crianças a brincar, ou a nadar, ou a comer, ou a chorar, etc.

Por: Felicidade N. Cherinda

2. The Boy Child

THE BOY CHILD
Sermon Text: Genesis 39:1-10

Introduction

Integrity comes from the fear of the Lord, and the fear of the Lord is learned from God's faithfulness. The life of Joseph in Egypt demonstrates this for us. It is a challenge to the adventures of youth, especially in the age of HIV/AIDS and sugar mummies. The Psalmist asks, "How can a young man keep his ways pure?" The response is, "By living according to your word" (Psalms 119:9). In spite of his misfortunes which turned out to be God's appointments, Joseph proved faithful to God and to his convictions.

This story is about many things. It is about powerful women and weak boys, mistresses and servants, and the vulnerability of house servants as sex objects, whether they are girls or boys. Many children are being sexually abused for ritual or cleansing purposes. In the process many children have contracted HIV/AIDS and other STDs. Sexual relationships need to be mutual and appropriate in terms of age, power relations and mental maturity.

We Listen to the Word of God

Put the following questions to the congregation:
- Who bought Joseph from the Ishmaelites?
- What caused Joseph to be trusted?
- What happened to the wealth of Potiphar on account of Joseph?
- What did Potiphar's wife say to Joseph?
- How did Joseph respond? Why?
- How does this story illustrate the vulnerability of house servants?
- What myths about manhood does this story go against?

We Apply the Word of God to Ourselves and the Congregation

WHAT CAN WE LEARN?
- That men of integrity say, "NO" to improper sex;
- That temptation happens;
- That there is always a way of escape; (Read I Corinthians 10:13)
- To run from temptation, is not to be a coward;
- Innocent suffering is possible in an evil world, but it needs to be remembered that in all things God works for good; (Read Romans 8:28)
- Women too can use their social and economic power to abuse boys or servants.

Consider also the following questions:
- How did Joseph maintain his integrity?
- How did Joseph influence his circumstances and how did his circumstances influence him?
- What remained constant in his response to his circumstances?
- What can we learn from Joseph in the way he dealt with his circumstances?

"The fear of the LORD is the beginning of wisdom." (Proverbs 9:10)

WHAT CAN WE CONFESS?
- Abuse of social power against the weak and vulnerable;
- Exposing the young to various dangers and diseases.

WHAT CAN WE BE THANKFUL FOR?
- Good moral training and upbringing;
- Acts of wisdom, courage and integrity.

WHAT CAN WE PRAY FOR?
- Children in vulnerable positions;
- Those who abuse children;
- Servants and immigrant workers in vulnerable positions.

WHAT CAN WE FEEL?
- Anger against abusers;
- Compassion for the abused;
- Admiration for those who resist temptation by showing integrity.

WHAT CAN WE BE?
- We can become sensitive and vigilant to the plight of the children, youth, servants and immigrants in our communities.

WHAT CAN WE DO?
- Work for children's rights and legal frameworks for their protection;
- Educate husbands on their sexual responsibilities towards their wives;
- Provide safe centres for victims to report to and be protected;
- Alert the community to the problem of child, servants and immigrant abuse;
- Promote sexual responsibility in church and society.

We Apply the Word of God to the Congregation/Society

- Can you identity similar scenarios taking place in our communities between masters/mistresses and servants, between doctors and patients, between teachers and pupils, between bosses and junior workers?
- What are you doing about children's exposure to pornography in your community?
- What are you doing about the myth of ritual cleansing for HIV/AIDS by using virgins?
- What is your congregation doing about sex in the media and commerce?
- Discuss some of the sexual myths related to men or women.

Song
When Upon Life's Billows, or **Count Your Blessings**

Prayer

There are many dangers on my life's pathway,
Send your light to enable me to recognize the danger.
Give me courage to face those I cannot avoid,
And wisdom to see the way of escape and use it.
Through Him who overcame temptation,
Though tried in every way,
He emerged without sin,
Even Jesus, the Christ. Amen

Suggested Objects/symbols/ideas: HIV/AIDS ribbon, cross, white cloth,
colour red for danger, etc.

By Augustine C. Musopule

The Boy Child
Sermon Text: Proverbs 4:1-23

Introduction

In many societies, the birth of a baby boy is characterized by much celebration, while that of a baby girl is muted (the speaker may cite local practices). In most African societies, the boy child is highly prized, as he is believed to ensure the survival of the lineage. Patriarchal values are also transmitted to the boy child through socialization.

It remains crucial for the boy child to receive gender sensitive training from an early age. In the HIV/AIDS context, the myth of male sexual conquest should be actively undermined. Furthermore, the boy child should be taught to play his part in providing care to the infected and affected. Emphasis should also be placed on the need for faithfulness in relationships.

We Listen to the Word of God

It is important that parents and guardians set aside time to impart words of wisdom to children. The text provides useful ethical guidelines for a young man. It calls upon him to value instructions if he is to have a long life. This acquisition of knowledge is particularly important in the light of HIV/AIDS. Young men and women require accurate information, alongside useful religious instructions.

We Apply the Word of God to Ourselves

WHAT CAN WE LEARN?
- Parents and guardians need to impart knowledge to their children;
- The boy child should be weaned from dangerous patriarchal values;
- Accurate knowledge and wisdom is crucial in the fight against HIV/AIDS;
- The boy child must be socialized to care, do house work and to value women.

WHAT DO WE HAVE TO CONFESS?
- Not finding time to teach children;
- Imparting dangerous values to the boy child in HIV/AIDS contexts;
- Passing on patriarchal values to the boy child.

WHAT CAN WE PRAY FOR?
- That God should empower us to bring up the boy child responsibly.

We Apply the Word of God to the Congregation

Get young men to stage a play where a young man gets distorted information and values about sexuality from his peers. Show the consequences. Then challenge the congregation to do its part.

Conclusion: A Word on Society

The image of a young man as a sexual predator is quite dominant in African societies. In addition, child rape, pornography and other vices have left young people vulnerable to HIV infection. Leaders at the different levels of society should act responsibly so that the boy child becomes an asset to society. The church should undertake to be an advocate for children's rights.

Song
Any local chorus that is child-friendly.

Prayer
God of Wisdom,
We pray for our young men,
That you may grant them discerning minds;
That they may hold on to your word;
That they may grow to express their sexuality responsibly.
Let our young men seek life-saving knowledge.
Let them grow to respect women.
Let them shun wicked and stifling systems.
Let them take care of the sick and lonely.
Accord them wisdom to protect the poor.
Nurture them to detest discrimination in all its forms.
Guide them to avoid the snare of drugs and the abuse of alcohol.

Mold them in the palm of your hand;
Pattern their lives after Jesus Christ.
Let them be truly humble and loving and responsible citizen
In Jesus' name we pray. Amen

Suggested Objects: Painting of a young man attending to a sick person.

By Ezra Chitando

3. The Girl Child

THE GIRL CHILD
Sermon Text: II Samuel 13

Prayer
By all

We are gathered together to affirm the humanity of the girl child. We celebrate the fact that the girl child was created in the image of God and is loved by God. We claim responsibility to protect the girl child and give her the opportunity to grow without fear of being abused by anyone. We pray for a safe environment that is created by all for the safety of the girl child. In Jesus Name. Amen

Song
Tswana

Tsholela Moya wa hau Jesu // (Pour your Spirit on us Jesus)
Tsholela Moya wa hau Jesu // (Pour your Spirit on us Jesus)
Dipilong rona Jesus // (Into our hearts, oh Jesus)
Tsholela Moya wa hau Jesus // (Pour your Spirit on us, Jesus)
(A popular Southern African Chorus)

Introduction

In general, cases of child abuse have increased in many parts of Africa in recent years, especially sexual abuse. The worst part of it is that there are more cases of infant abuse. This high rate can be linked to the myth that when an HIV positive person sleeps with a virgin, they are cured from the virus. Unfortunately, not enough is being done to expose this as a rumor. Child abuse is also on the increase because people concerned have taken a position of silence. Both men and women know that children are being sexually abused, but for one reason or another keep quite about it. We cannot emphasize enough the importance of breaking the silence.

The process of curbing child abuse involves everyone: parents, other members of the family, teachers, doctors and nurses, the police, social workers, the legal system and the church.

We Listen to the Word of God

We read II Samuel 13. The leader or a member of the congregation can read the story. This story can also be dramatized.

DETAILS OF THE TEXT

The characters of the story are as follows:

> **Tamar** is the main character in the story. She is the daughter of King David and Maacah of Geshur. She is a full sister of Absolom and half sister of Amnon. She is the object of Amnon's lust. She willingly goes to take care of a sick brother. Out of trust, she agrees to prepare a meal for her brother Ammon in his quarters. When she saw that she was in danger, she tried to reason with him, by telling him that rape is wrong according to their faith and culture. She is even willing to offer an alternative; marriage between sister and brother through negotiations with their father King David. Despite her resistance, she is raped, because he does not listen to her. She is thrown out. She did not keep quiet about it. She wept loudly, put ashes on her head, and tore the nice clothes that symbolised her virginity. By her actions, she let the whole of the king's compound know that she had been raped. Her whole future was ruined on that day, because we are told she spent the rest of her life as a lonely person in Absolom's home.

> **Amnon** was the first born son of King David and Ahinoam. Amnon was the most likely person to become the next king of Israel. He lusted after his sister, Tamar to the point of plotting to rape her. With the help of a friend, he succeeded in raping his sister. Immediately, he developed a hatred for his sister, and threw her out of his house. Two years later, his brother Absolom killed him for raping Tamar.

> **Jonadab** was a cousin and close friend of Amnon. He was a bad influence on Amnon because he is the one who planned the raping of his other cousin, Tamar. He believed that a son of a king should not be denied, even if it is at the expense of another person's life. He did not care what would happen to his cousin, Tamar. All he wanted was for Ammon to manifest that he had the power to get whatever he wanted.

> **King David** was the king of Israel. He was also a family man, the father of Amnon, Absolom, Tamar and the uncle of Jonadab. In this story, David is a father who is unable to come to the defense of his daughter; Tamar after his son raped her. We are told that when he heard the story he was furious, but did nothing.

> **Absalom** was the third born son of King David. He took his sister into his house to stay with him after she was raped. He told his sister not to take the abuse seriously because her brother did it. However, two years later he revenged the rape of Tamar by killing Amnon. He also named his daughter after Tamar.

We Apply the Word of God to Ourselves

WHAT CAN WE LEARN?

- That Tamar was a girl of integrity. She protested violence against women. Her major crime was that she was born a beautiful woman.
- Sometimes women and girl children are not safe from rape, even in a God fearing home and among people that are supposed to be trusted.
- Rape is not induced by what a woman is wearing, the place where she is, or the class that she belongs to. It can happen to any woman and child at any time and anywhere – including the safety of their homes.
- The character of Amnon teaches us that rapists are found in all classes and races.
- Jonadab teaches us what Paul said in I Corinthians 15: 33, that 'bad company corrupts'.
- The silence of David reminds us of the saying that the men who rape women and children are a few, but those who are silent about it are many. It is the silence that motivates the perpetrators to continue the abuse.
- The initial silence of Absalom who did not confront Amnon, Jonadab and King David, tells us that justice delayed is justice denied. His revenge indicates that the whole family was wounded and needed healing.

WHAT DO WE HAVE TO CONFESS?

- We have not created a safe environment for our daughters even in our homes;
- We have kept silent, even when we know of the rape of the girl child that we live with;
- We have delayed acting on a rape case for fear of exposing another loved one, or to protect our own financial venerability at the expense of our girl children;
- We have not preached against rape or violence against women;
- We have endangered raped children by not taking them to the hospital.

WHAT CAN WE BE THANKFUL FOR?

- Jesus heals traumatized girl children who have been raped;
- Even the perpetrators of rape can confess their sins and be forgiven by God, though they may suffer the consequences of their actions;
- The many NGOs and church related organizations who are blowing the whistle on rapists;
- The new laws in some countries that have been set up to protect girl children from rape.

WHAT CAN WE PRAY FOR?

- For the many girl children who are still being raped, that by the grace of God someone will come to their defense and they will be able to come out from the situation of rape;
- The many women who are having marital problems because of their childhood rape experience, that they will seek inner healing;
- The rapist to come to the realization that what they are doing is wrong and to stop;
- A communal effort to combat rape;
- Severe sentences to deter would be rapists;
- More facilities to be made available to counsel rape victims and perpetrators;
- Better hospital facilities and medicines.

We Apply the Word of God to the Congregation

WHAT CAN WE FEEL?
- Sad, that rape cases are found even in Christian homes;
- Sorry for the girls and women whose future is ruined because of a rape experience, especially when HIV infection is a result of the rape;
- Ashamed for keeping quiet when rape was happening with our knowledge;
- Anger toward the rapists, but also compassion when they seek help.

WHAT CAN WE BE?
- A community that girls can trust and confide in;
- A healing community for victims and perpetrators.

WHAT CAN WE DO?
- Preach against violence against children and women. We need to break the chains of silence.
- Provide shelter for victims of rape. Let us begin by creating an atmosphere of trust so that the victims can have the courage to talk about it. We are the hands and feet of Jesus. Let the compassion of Jesus come out in us, to provide care for those who are victims.
- We also need to declare a zero tolerance zone for any form of sexual abuse.
- We need to be open enough to accommodate the perpetrators of abuse. Confronting them alone will not solve the problem, they also need to be led to deliverance. We know Jesus as the one who delivers us from all forms of evil.
- We need to give back to people the sense of integrity and a purpose for life.
- Dispel the myth that having sex with a virgin cures people from HIV.
- Set up strong counseling services in church.

We Apply the Word of God to the Society

The problem of rape and all abuse is a result of a sick society that has not connected itself to the authority of God. When Adam and Eve rebelled against God, sin entered the world. All kinds of evil began to manifest. Abuse is one kind of those evils. We thank God for Jesus Christ who came to redeem humanity from evil. Therefore all those who repent of their sins and accept the Lordship of Jesus, become new creatures. The old life of evil is taken away from them, and a new nature is created in them. The new nature in Jesus needs to be nurtured on a daily basis, so that one does not loose focus and manifest things of the flesh. It is in Christ that men and women develop a relationship of respect and trust. This is where one finds true love that protects the other from all that is harmful. In Christ we show that we love God by the way we treat others. A person who abuses another has lost a sense of dignity and integrity.

Prayer
By all:
We thank you God because you identify with the oppressed. You were there when Tamar was raped and you identify with all the girls and women who identify with Tamar's experience.

Thank you for requesting us abused women and children to surrender to you our painful experience, so that you can cover us with your healing hands.

Thank you for exchanging our painful experience with your free gift of love that will make us a new creation.

Thank you God, because you are the healer of those of us here who identify with Amnon, Jonadab, King David and Absalom, as families torn by sexual abuse. Thank you for calling us to genuine repentance that leads to the forgiveness of sins. We ask for will power not to do it again, but to completely turn around and start a new life of building healthy relationships with women and girls in our homes and community.

We declare Jesus as the healer of our families and communities from the spirit of abuse and deliberate infection of each other with HIV. Amen

Song (Zulu)
Ukuhlabelela, kuyamthokozisa // (To sing makes the one)
Odabukileyo hlabelela // (Who is downcast happy)
Sithi: Bonga, bonga bonga…// (We say: thank you…)
Njenge 'nyoni endle // (Like a bird in the veld)
Hlabelela // (Sing!)

Zonk'izingelosi
Ziyayibon' Inkosi // (All the angels thank the Lord)
Zibong'umusa wayo // (Thank God for mercy)
Hlabelela! // (Sing!)
(A Popular South African Chorus)

Benediction
May the healing power of God surround you all the days of your life. May you pass on the power of healing to your home and community. May others experience the healing power of God through your actions and presence.

Symbols/objects/ideas: Play games that show trust; find examples of people who need healing from abuse or as abusers; water to wash hands as a symbol of new life; pictures of water, or mountains that portray the healing power of God, and musical instruments.

By Isabel Apawo Phiri

170

SERVICE FOCUSING ON THE GIRL CHILD
Sermon Text: Judges 11:34-40

Prayer

Lord, we thank you for the gift of children, especially girl children. In this service we ask you to enable us to focus on them. Through this service, we appeal to you to remind us that children are not our possessions in the sense that we possess other things. We thank you for the joy they bring into our lives. So we lift children up and commit them to your love and care, even as we pray that you will make us worthy adults and parents. All this we ask in the name of Jesus Christ our Lord, Amen.

Song

An appropriate song focusing either on children in general, or on girl children in particular may be sung.

Introduction

It is an open secret, that alongside the elderly, children are one of the most vulnerable groups in society. Governments and societies often treat children as if they were dispensable. The forcible and illegal use of children in many of the senseless wars in Africa is a case in point. While there have been strong movements in defense of the rights of Blacks, women and to some extent, the elderly, there has been no sustained movement for child rights, equal or comparable in sophistication and articulation to, for example, the feminist movement. This too is sign of the extent to which children remain vulnerable. It is especially the girl children who are at the bottom of the pile. It is girl children who are the main target of child sex rings and cross border trafficking in women and children. There are many other, less dramatic ways in which girl children continue to receive the shorter end of the stick. In many cultures, the manner in which girls and boys are socialized means that girls are groomed to become servants. This has direct bearing on HIV/AIDS incidence among girl children. Powerless and at the mercy of men, girl children have no choice when it comes to sexual matters.

We Listen to the Word of God

We read Judges 11
DETAILS OF THE TEXT
To understand this strange sounding passage, it is important to read the eleventh chapter of the book of Judges from the beginning. Effectively, Jephthah was a mercenary whose reward was headship. Under siege, and humiliating and repeated attacks by the Ammonites, the leaderless and kingless Israelites appealed for help to Jephthah, whose skill and strength as warrior was well-known. "What is in it for me," was the first question that Jephthah asked them? "You will become our head and leader?" This answer worked like magic. Not only did the elders play on Jephthah's ambitions for political office, but they also happened to know his sorry and sad background, and sought to cash in on his deep-seated feelings of inadequacy and his deep longing for acceptance. He was, after all, the son of a sex worker, born out of wedlock and chased away from his home by his father's legitimate children. He was, therefore, not only ambitious, but he also bore the emotional and psychological scars of derision and rejection for being the illegitimate

171

son of a sex worker. When the people who used to taunt him, approach him for help, he cannot but think that at long last he may find genuine acceptance and belonging with his father's people.

Such is the depth of the scars in his soul, and such is his ambition for political office, that he makes a rash and poorly thought out wager with God. "If you give the Ammonites into my hands, whatever comes out of the door of my house to meet me when I return in triumph from the Ammonites will be the Lord's, and I will sacrifice it as a burnt offering." Such was his ambition for political office and his sense of personal inadequacy, that he made this thoughtless pledge to God. Knowing fully well that he had only one child, a girl child, he might have guessed that either his wife or daughter or both would come and meet him if he returned in triumph from war.

In pursuit of his ambition and in an attempt to resolve his psychological problems, Jephthah renders his wife and daughter dispensable. On his way from and to glory, he brings about the death of his own daughter. She dies in order to keep the honour of her father, and in order for her father's ambition to be fulfilled. She dies because her father has unresolved psychological problems. She dies so her father may become leader of Gilead for six years.
How many girl children are HIV positive because a father or an uncle has sought to use them either in his way to or from perceived glory? How many girl children orphaned by HIV/AIDS have fallen foul to the unbridled ambitions of relatives, who step in to claim and control their deceased parents' assets?

We Apply the Word of God to Ourselves

WHAT CAN WE LEARN?
- That children, especially girl children, are often treated as cogs in the machine of men's and society's political and economic ambitions;
- That children are often treated as if they were dispensable;
- That children are often the victims of unresolved psychological and political problems of their parents, and of the societies in which they live;
- As the most vulnerable group, girl children often bear the brunt of the HIV/AIDS epidemic, either as they contract the disease by being forced to have sex, or as they have to care for siblings after the death of their parents.

WHAT DO WE HAVE TO CONFESS?
- That we render our children dispensable;
- That society often makes children secondary to, and servants of, society's ambitions;
- That girl children continue to be the most vulnerable members of society;
- That we have neglected concerted church action in defense of girl children.

WHAT CAN WE BE THANKFUL FOR?
- For the gift of girl children;
- For parents and societies which care about and for children;
- For the resilience of girl children and their amazing community roles in HIV/AIDS ravaged communities.

WHAT CAN WE PRAY FOR?
- For girl children in Africa and all over the world;
- For girl children affected or infected with HIV/AIDS;
- For girl children taking care of parents dying of HIV/AIDS;
- For girl children caring for siblings and grandparents after the death of their own parents.

We Apply the Word of God to the Congregation

WHAT CAN WE FEEL?
- We should feel remorse at the manner in which society treats girl children;
- We should feel hopeful for those girl children who are caring for either dying parents, or siblings after the death of parents.

WHAT CAN WE BE?
- We can become parents to orphaned girl children;
- We can make the church a home for abused and orphaned girl children.

Conclusion: A Word to Society

The plight of girl children is a serious one in our times. They who ought to be our last defense against the deadly plague of HIV/AIDS, are nevertheless rendered the most vulnerable to it and other menaces of our times. Whereas the plight of child soldiers in some African wars has been highlighted, what happens to girl children in those situations has seldom been mentioned. Churches must arise and do something to save and defend the girl child.

Prayer of Commitment:
The girl child is made in your image and likeness. Her body is a temple of your Holy Spirit. Help us to remember and protect the rights of the girl child. Amen

Song
Thuma Mina

Symbols/objects and commitments: Beads, dolls, clothes.

By Tinyiko S. Maluleke

4. Youth

Youth Service
Sermons Text: Ecclesiastes 11:7-12, 8

Introduction

Statistical evidence tells us that youths between the ages 15-29 are the most vulnerable to the HIV/AIDS pandemic. Most of the people in Sub-Saharan Africa who are infected by the virus fall within this age bracket. It is therefore difficult to be a young African. The innocence of youth has been taken away by this deadly disease. Growing up in the era of HIV/AIDS is dangerous. It is very unsafe to be a young African, because the probability of being 'a statistic' is very high.

African youths used to undergo traditional rituals such as female and male initiation schools, where they were taught about human sexuality. These institutions are no longer there. Many of them live in poverty, and often find themselves being lured by people with money for casual sex. It is especially girls who are sexually abused by older men 'to cleanse' themselves from HIV/AIDS. So the service needs to take on board these realities.

We Listen to the Word of God

DETAILS OF THE TEXT
- These words are an admonition to both the young and the old on how to live.
- The preacher reminds us that we all die at some point, and when we die we shall be judged by whatever we did while living.
- A few things to note are that young people should enjoy their youth, what does this mean?
- Youth should remember their creator, and we should all know that we shall grow old and weak, and we shall die and return to the dust of the earth.

We Apply the Word of God to Ourselves and the Congregation

Churches have an obligation to create the right environment for young people to enjoy their faith, their membership to the church, and their youth. Over the years the church has made it difficult for youths to experience freedom and joy in the church. The church also has the responsibility to advocate for the rights of youth. This requires that church leaders should be knowledgeable about the different conventions and charters that enshrine the rights of youths. Among these is the African Charter for Children.

WHAT DO WE LEARN?
Admonition is something that is rare in many communities these days. HIV/AIDS has ravaged the social fabric of African societies, and as a result the extended family system has been terribly weakened. However, we have to find other systems through which we can help young people to 'remember the Creator in their youth,' and to avoid the pitfalls that lie in the way.

We also have to help our young people to find the right ways to 'enjoy their youths'. Many young people use drugs, abuse alcohol and are involved with gangsters as a way of 'having fun'. This is not what the preacher is advocating for when he says 'enjoy your youth'. It is important that whatever the youths do, they are admonitioned to remember their creator as well.

WHAT CAN WE CONFESS?
We need to confess that:
- The Church has over the years not given the youths space to exercise their faith in Christ;
- The church does not provide youth friendly services, such as education on adolescent reproductive health, recreational activities and open 'spaces' to get a youth agenda going;
- The failure of the church to provide mentoring, admonition and guidance to youths.

WHAT CAN WE BE THANKFUL FOR?
- Although the statistics of HIV/AIDS are horrifying, it is important to remember that more than 70% of people living in Sub-Saharan Africa are HIV negative. We should celebrate this and seek to raise that figure
- We thank God for youth leaders and activists who are involved in youth activities that are about combating HIV/AIDS
- We rejoice in what the churches are doing to enable their youths to explore their faith freely, and to enjoy their youth.

WHAT CAN WE PRAY FOR?
"An audacious dream"
These words can be said to a rap tune.

I dream of a world where the youth are free,
Free to play with each other without fear,
Free to touch, tickle and to embrace,
Free to be themselves and be respected for that.

I dream of a world where the young blossom,
Where potential is harnessed and realized,
Where people's efforts are rewarded,
And where one can fly to reach the sky

I dream of a church that is inclusive,
Where I am not the church of tomorrow,
Where I am permitted to sing my own tune,
Where I am belong in my own right.

I dream of a world without HIV/AIDS,
I dream of a kaleidoscope of African youths,
Who sing a song of praise and not shed tears,
I dream of life in fullness and no more death.

Song

Seek ye first the kingdom of God,
And the righteousness,
Then all these things will be
Given unto you,

Alleluia, alleluia. (3x)

Ask and it shall be given to you,
Seek and you shall find,
Knock and the door shall be
Opened unto you,

Alleluia, alleluia. (3x)

Man does not live by bread alone,
But by every bread,
That proceeds from mouth of God,

Alleluia, alleluia. (3x)
(Anonymous)

Suggested objects/symbols/ideas: Use newspaper cuttings and put them in a collage to show some of the things that are happening to young people in the community.

By Moiseraele P. Dibeela

5. Parents and Parenthood

THE ROLE OF A PARENT
Sermon Text: I Samuel 2:2-17

Introduction

The role of parents has become increasingly difficult in our changing society. The cohesiveness of the traditional extended family is now falling apart in Botswana and other parts of Africa. In fact, a recent workshop questioned the definition of the family, as many feel that it is not so easy to define anymore, and changes all the time. In the past, the whole village did the parenting of child. The parents, uncles and aunts, the neighbors, teachers, traditional leaders and community leaders like church ministers, each had a role to play. Urbanization broke this concept of parenting. With Botswana having the highest rate of HIV /AIDS in Sub-Saharan Africa, the number of orphans rises daily. The load of parenting has become overwhelming in every family. Western influences have also had an impact on the lives of both parents and children. This brings in attitudes like individualism and materialism, which make people care less about the other. The cultural gap between the children and parents is also growing, which gives rise to more conflict and misunderstandings. This again could be contributed to external influences.

We Listen to the Word of God

DETAILS OF THE TEXT
The text introduces us to two families, Hannah's family and Eli's family. Samuel, Hannah's son faithfully performed his tasks under Eli, grew in spiritual stature and developed a relationship with God that grew in power and intimacy. Then, there are the sons of Eli; Hophni and Phinenas. These two seemed to drift further and further from God, and the teachings with which they were brought up.

There are two important lessons for me in reading this story. The first important one is to take responsibility as a parent by 'handing over' one's child to God. Hannah believed that God gave Samuel to her, and therefore she needed to hand back that child to God. This means handing over our children through prayer, baptism, Sunday school, and confirmation class and youth fellowship. Through these, the child could be nurtured in the body of Christ to grow spiritually.

The second lesson, for me, is that often we as parents do not make time to actually raise the children and teach them right from wrong. Eli might have been so busy in doing his work as priest that he failed as a parent to teach his children about the God that he so faithfully served. His sons therefore saw what Eli did more as mere rituals, rather than a true relationship with God. His children did not learn from Eli the meaning of sacrifice, devotion and service unto God. It could also be that there developed a cultural gap between Eli and his sons, as they grew older. This resulted into them not appreciating their father's relationship with God. Eli too, was seen to have failed in his role as parent as 'he did not restrain them', (I Samuel 3:13), and therefore brought punishment on his household.

We Apply the Word of God to Ourselves

WHAT CAN WE LEARN?
- That we need to bring our children up in God's household;
- That we need to pray for our children.

WHAT DO WE HAVE TO CONFESS?
- That we are weak most of the time in correcting and restraining our children for the wrongs that they do;
- That we do not bring our children to God in prayer or raise them in God's household;
- That the children are abused within our families;
- That we have not done enough to protect children from HIV/AIDS.

WHAT CAN WE BE THANKFUL FOR?
- For the many children who, like Samuel, grow spiritually and intimately in their relationship with God;
- For the families who provide protection, time and discipline into bringing their children up to fear God;
- For many children who are not infected by HIV/AIDS.

WHAT CAN WE PRAY FOR?
- For single mothers who struggle to raise their children without support from fathers;
- For the disintegrating family life through which children have no role models and guidance;
- For the many children out living on the street, those who are abused from a young age, children who are in prisons, and orphans who have nobody to take care of them;
- For child- headed homes, who have lost their parents to HIV/AIDS.

We Apply the Word of God to our Church/Society

WHAT CAN WE DO?
- Conduct parenting courses to help parents to improve their relationships with their children;
- Set up youth groups and children's groups to help children understand their contribution to the family and God's teachings;
- Improve Sunday school and youth programmes to be relevant to the family and the problems experienced in families;
- Provide support groups for parents who find parenting difficult;
- Train and encourage families to adopt and care for the orphans;
- For youth to start homework help for orphans.

Song
The leader may choose any appropriate song.

Prayer

God our mother and father,
You graciously look upon us and take care of us.
You cloth us, feed us, and guide us with truth and wisdom.

We bring to your altar all parents. We often
Do not have all that it takes to raise our children.
We pray that you might help us to fulfill our role
With the love and discipline it deserves.
Make us stronger, wiser, more loving, in Jesus name.
Amen

Suggested Symbols/ideas: Drawings of huts, families.

By Cheryl Dibeela

SERVICE FOR SINGLE PARENTS
Suggested Passage: Matthew 15:21-28

Opening Prayer of Thanksgiving

Leader 1: Father and Mother God,
We thank you as single parents, especially as single mothers.
We thank you, for you are the Father and Mother of our families.

All: We thank you, for the stone that was rejected has become the cornerstone.

Leader 2: We thank you for Ishmael, Hagar's child,
Who became the ancestor of a great nation.
We thank, for you are the Father and Mother of single mothers' children.

All: We thank you, for the stone that was rejected has become the cornerstone.

Leader 3: We thank you for Obed, the child of Ruth,
Who became the great ancestor of David.
We thank you for you are the Father and Mother of child-headed homes.

All: We thank you, for the stone that was rejected has become the cornerstone.

Leader 4: We thank you for Solomon, the child of Bathsheba,
Who became a great king of wisdom.
We thank you, for you are the Father and Mother of single
Parent families.

All: We thank you that the stone that was rejected has become the cornerstone.

Leader 5: We thank you for Jesus, the child of Mary,
Who became the savior of the world.
We thank you, for you are the Father and Mother of grandmothers'
children

All: We thank you, for the stone that was rejected has become the cornerstone.

179

Introduction

In many societies and cultures, single parenting is increasingly becoming common for various reasons. Urban-rural migration, labor migration, political and economic upheavals, globalization, unemployment and HIV/AIDS are among many other factors that increasingly put pressure on the family, particularly the marriage institution. Often mothers and grandmothers, by virtue of their gendered roles as nurturers, carry the burdens of raising children alone. Nonetheless, single mothers and their parents still suffer discrimination from their communities and churches. It is important for the church leaders to see single parenting as part of our reality, our societies, our world and our churches and to offer a ministry that affirms single parents and their children.

Towards this end, the above prayer highlights that in salvation history, God does not discriminate against any child, in fact God blesses the rejected stone. In the reading that follows, the struggle of single parents is brought to the fore, and the need for the church to hear their cries and to support them is underlined. While almost all parents are particularly living with uncertainty for their children, the situation of single parents is even worse in the HIV/AIDS era. For example, how does a single parent earn a living if one of her children is sick and needs home-based care or if the parent is sick them self? Yet HIV/AIDS has also brought forth new types of families to the fore: child-headed households, the grandmother-headed households and the single father.

We Listen to the Word of God

Reading the text: Matthew 15:21-28
DETAILS OF THE TEXT
Verses 21:
➢ The setting of the story is provided, stating the geographical place of the story.

Verse 22:
➢ A new character is introduced. She is a Canaanite woman. Note that she comes to Jesus seeking help alone, unaccompanied. Given the culture of that time, this strongly suggests that she was a single parent.

➢ Highlight that she comes to Jesus in desperation: she starts off shouting, calling for help on behalf of her severely possessed daughter. Underline that she asks for mercy: "Have mercy on me," she desperately appeals to Jesus.

Verse 23:
➢ Note that both Jesus and the disciples do not respond to the woman's call for help. "Jesus did not answer her at all," and the disciples said, "Send her away."

➢ Note that the woman was following them shouting for help. Put the question to the congregation if we sometimes ignore single parents who desperately need our help.

Verse 24:
➢ Jesus gives a reason for his silence: his ministry is exclusively for the Israelites. He cannot attend to the needs of Canaanite child. It is an ethnic-based response. Do we sometimes discriminate on the basis of ethnicity?

Verse 25:
➢ Note that the woman disregards their resistance. She insists. She comes forward and kneels before Jesus and states her plea, "Lord, help me."

Verse 26:
➢ Jesus finally speaks to her, stating the reasons for his silence. He does not think that Israelite children's bread should be thrown to the dogs (Canaanite children).

➢ Note the differentiation, some are children, others are dogs. Who are the dogs and who are the children in your context, church, family and community?

➢ Highlight how Jesus speaks of healing as children's bread. What is the link between food and health?

Verse 27:
➢ Underline that the woman still persists, searching for help for her sick child. She assures Jesus that she does not seek to deny Israelites children of the bread, nonetheless other children also need bread; they need healing. She thus asks for crumbs. Jesus grants it to her on the basis of her persistent faith.

➢ Underline that we need to persistently insist for the needs of all children.

➢ Of note here is the woman's persistence and Jesus' willingness to reconsider his initial position, when confronted by another truth—namely, all children are children. All children deserve health and bread.

We Apply the Word of God to Ourselves

WHAT CAN LEARN?
• That all children deserve bread on the table;
• That many single parents are seeking our help;
• To be persistent parents in search for our children's health;
• That we can share the bread of our children with children of single parents.

WHAT DO WE HAVE TO CONFESS?
Prayer of confession:
• We confess that we have not always listened to the cries of single parents;
• We have not always seen all children as equal;
• We confess that we still refer to children from different ethnic groups and single parents as dogs, and deny them the space at the table and bread;

- We confess that our discriminatory look on single mothers and their children means that they become more vulnerable to HIV/AIDS. Help us to hear their cries and to welcome them at our table fellowship. Amen

WHAT CAN WE BE THANFUL FOR?
- That many single mothers are committed to the wellbeing of their children;
- That Jesus is not afraid to change his mind about a Canaanite child;
- That Jesus is brought to share bread of healing with all children.

WHAT CAN WE PRAY FOR?
- That all children, should be treated equally;
- That single mothers should be heard and their needs met in the society;
- That our churches should become parenting churches.

We Apply the Word of God to the Congregation

WHAT CAN WE BE?
- An inclusive church to single parents and grandmothers;
- A welcoming church to children of single parents and of all ethnic groups;
- A prophetic church on the rights of single parents and their children.

WHAT CAN WE DO?
- Set up an services that highlight our support for single parents;
- Run workshops on single parenting;
- Start a programmatic response for child and grandmother headed households.

Conclusion: A Word on Society

While the society may neglect the needs of single parents, or look down upon them, the Christian church must challenge itself to listen to them and to walk with them. In the HIV/AIDS era, the burden of single parents calls a church to become a parenting church.
In particular, the emergence of new types of families: the child and the grandmother headed homes, underlines the need for the church to develop a ministry of parenting with single parents. It also calls for a church that undertakes advocacy for single parents and their children.

Song
Choose an appropriate song.

Closing Prayer
Creator God, in a world of broken families and societies,
In a world of immense labor immigration and displaced people,
In a world of economic and political upheavals,
In a world of globalization and diseases, especially HIV/AIDS,
Many are raising children as single parents.

Loving and caring God, we thank you for you love for all children,
We thank you for to the single mothers, for you are the Father to their children,
And to single fathers, you are the Mother to their children,
To the grandparents and child headed household, you are the Father and Mother
to their orphaned children. Amen

Objects/symbols/ideas: Zimbabwean/Kenyan stone abstract carvings indicating unity; Mary with Jesus/Mother with child poster; Proverbs: It takes a village to raise a child; *mmangwana o tshwara thipa ka fa bogaleng* (a mother holds a knife by its cutting edge).

By Musa W. Dube

6. Men and Fatherhood

MEN AND THEIR ROLE IN COMMUNITY
Sermon Text: Genesis 19:1-11

Prayer
In this service oh Lord, we wish to commend men before you. We live in a world where masculinity has become abused and distorted. In many parts of the world, men are socialized to believe in force and domination. In many cultures men are brought up to suppress and disown their feelings. African men are no exception. We implore you to journey with us as we explore alternative ways of being men. We pray that you will give us the resources to become men of God and to bring our sons up as such. All this we pray in the name of Jesus Christ, our Lord. Amen

Song
An appropriate song on manhood or cooperation between men and women may be sung.

Introduction

There is a crisis of masculinity. There is a crisis of what it means to be a man. The symptoms of this crisis are to be seen in the predominant images of masculinity in our cultures. In many cultures, men are brought up to be and treated as chiefs to be pampered, to rule and to command. In various ways men are taught and socialized into believing in force and power over. The HIV/AIDS crisis has brought matters to a head. If men continue to dominate, coerce and to believe that that is what it means to be men, then HIV/AIDS prevention campaigns will come to naught. For in these contexts women have no right and possibility of control for their choices and their bodies. Although seldom remarked, the truth is that women are the worst victims of the many violent wars going on in the world. The raping of women is both an old and contemporary weapon of war.

183

We Listen to the Word of God

We read from Genesis 19:1-11
DETAILS OF THE TEXT
There has been much unwarranted controversy - especially on the subject of homosexuality - based on this passage. For some it is a passage that proves that homosexuality is wrong. Yet others argue that if anything, this story points to widespread practice of homosexuality. Lot is shocked not by the fact and nature of the demand of the men who are banging at the door, but by its violent intentions directed at guests and strangers, some would say. Lot displays no shock at the intended homosexual nature of the sex being demanded as such. Others point out that this is really a story of rape - threatened rape - first and foremost. I concur. Secondly it is a story of violence, masculine violence. Hence the pathetic but spine-chilling offer of Lot: "I have two daughters who have never slept with a man. Let me bring them out to you, and you can do what you like with them." At this stage it becomes clear that this is a story of men at war among and between themselves - a war in which women can be thoughtlessly used as ransom and as forms of comfort. This then is a shameful story of perverse manhood flirting - as usual - with violence as a means of communication, relationship and self-assertion. It is a story about men seeking to assert power over other men and doing so in complete disregard to the welfare of women - indeed using women in the process. It is the story of a sick manly contest between Lot and his neighbors - which must have antecedents before the arrival of the two guests. This is the story of manhood gone mad in its pursuit for power and dominance. To come to our own context it is important for us to note that HIV/AIDS thrives on violence and distorted notions of masculinity.

We Apply the Word of God and to Ourselves

WHAT CAN WE LEARN?
- That there is a link between distorted notions of masculinity and violence;
- There is a link between rape and violence, indeed that rape is not about sex but about violence;
- That women are often victims in the battles of men for power and control;
- That there is a link between the distorted notions of masculinity, violence and the spread of HIV/AIDS.

WHAT DO WE HAVE TO CONFESS?
- We confess that our societies, in various ways, continue to socialize men for power and dominance;
- We confess that distorted notions of masculinity make victims of women and put the world constantly on the road to self-destruction.

WHAT CAN WE BE THANKFUL FOR?
- We can be thankful for some men who are already seeking alternative ways of being men, relating with other men, and relating with women.
- We can be thankful that though Jesus Christ came as a man, he nevertheless related to both men and women in life affirming rather than violent ways.

WHAT CAN WE PRAY FOR?
- We pray for the conversion of men from violence to love;
- We pray for the conversion of relations between men and men so that masculinity is redefined in terms of love rather than power over others;
- We pray for the conversion of relations between men and women, so that they may relate as self-respecting equals without need to resort to violence and coercion;
- We pray that our churches may become schools and factories for these kinds of men.

We Apply the Word of God to the Congregation

WHAT CAN WE FEEL?
- As men, we should feel remorse at the centrality of violence and coercion in the manner in which we relate to one another and to women;
- We should feel sad that society continues to socialize men and women for violent and unequal relationships.

WHAT CAN WE BE?
- We can be inspired by the example of Jesus in the manner in which he conducted his manhood, and in the manner in which he related both to men and women.

WHAT CAN WE DO?
- We should propose concrete ways in which our churches can focus on the training and retraining men from violence, to mutuality and respect for others.
- We should explain the link between rape and violence and the spread of HIV/AIDS.

Conclusion: A Word to Society

Men must be taught different and new ways of being men. This cannot be left to Hollywood and growing militarization. We have to find ways in which men can be taught and re-taught love and relationship. If this is not done, we have little chance of stemming the tide of the HIV/AIDS pandemic.

Prayer of Commitment
Ask one individual to make a prayer.

Song
Choose any appropriate song.

Symbols/objects/ideas and commitments: A doll, a child, a heart, etc.

By Tinyiko S. Maluleke

MEN AND THE USE OF POWER
Sermon Text: Mark 9:33-36

Introduction

It is difficult to talk about power in patriarchal Africa, without talking about masculinity. Masculinity throughout the ages has been, and still is, equated with power; both physical and emotional; as well as the power of authority, and the power to lead and to make decisions. This is evident within all spheres of life, politics, the home and sadly in the Church too. This masculine power almost always exerts supremacy that is negative, yet it is always encouraged by society as a positive attribute. Some of the negative examples, including sexual harassment perpetrators at work, are men. This abuse of power is also found in child abuse, domestic violence and rape. This very domineering abuse of power that has contributed to the transmission of HIV/AIDS. Decision-making on sexual issues is left to men; whether or not he wants to use condoms. This has implications for the care-giving role, as well as such characteristics needed to fulfill the responsibility of career are not associated with male authority.

Women, on the other hand, especially those fortunate enough to occupy leadership positions within society, are often encouraged to adopt these male characteristics. If they don't, then they are viewed as 'weak or emotional'. These characteristics in society are referred to as negative attributes. They are seen to lack confidence and assertiveness. Women and men are socialized by society to accept the dominance of men. This has led to women not being seen as capable of leading, making decisions and accepting positions of power when men are around. These are all factors that affect women negatively with HIV/AIDS, as they are most of the times not decision-makers within sexual relationships.

We Listen to the Word of God

DETAILS OF THE TEXT

It is ironic that this question of greatness and power had to be posed by male disciples. In spite of what Jesus taught about servanthood, his disciples were still preoccupied with power. Commentators believe that the disciples' failure and lack of understanding typify the patterns of successive generations, who persist in setting their minds on such human things. This is true and visible even among women's conversations and livelihood today, although it is still dominant among men. The disciples were equally caught up with their own questions of greatness, and slow to understand what Jesus stood for.

Jesus is once again the revolutionary character, as he sets new categories of 'greatness'. He uses a child, the most marginalized member in our society, the most humble and sometimes the most ignored, as having the lowest social status. Jesus in using the example of a child, also proposes alternatives of power: the power to care, love and embrace those who are different. Jesus, a male, could have easily rested in the comfort that men experienced at the time, but he did not. We are challenged, just as Jesus brought his disciples to a stand still, 'And he sat down and called the twelve' (v. 35). This, seems to be an indication that he regarded this as an important issue.

We ought to bring life to a stand still, for males and females to set new standards of power especially in this HIV/AIDS context. We need Christ's standards of overturning the norm.

We Apply the Word of God to Ourselves

WHAT CAN WE LEARN?
- That our concept of power is not Jesus' concept;
- The power of humility and lowliness;
- That there are more important things in life than power of status, control, etc.;
- That Christian power is the power to love and care.

WHAT DO WE HAVE TO CONFESS?
- That we often strive towards power for importance and dominance;
- That a lot of hurt is caused through abuse of power;
- That as men we have not used our power to prevent HIV/AIDS;
- That as men we have failed to care and nurse those who have HIV/AIDS.

WHAT CAN WE BE THANKFUL FOR?
- For Jesus' example;
- For the homes, work places and churches in which power is shared and not abused;
- For many people who humbly take care of those who need it;
- For the opportunity to emulate Jesus.

WHAT CAN WE PRAY FOR?
- That those who abuse power might experience a time of reflection;
- That men and women together accept servant-hood;
- That the HIV/AIDS era, men should use their power to love and care for their wives and children and protect them from infection.

We Apply the Word of God to our Church/Society

WHAT CAN WE DO?
- Teach on aspects of gender and how power has an influence;
- Teach boys and girls from an early age about Jesus' concept of power;
- Teach men and women about HIV/AIDS and power in the society;
- Discuss on how men can make a difference in the HIV/AIDS struggle.

The following prayer could be used during this service.

Prayer

Congregation:	God who is the greatest among us?
Leader:	Not the man that has only revenge in mind, just to kill and to maim, But the one whoever receives a child in my name, receives me.
Congregation:	God who is the greatest among us?
Leader:	Not the man who makes and obeys laws which reduce others to a

	lower status than themselves. But whoever receives a child in my name receives me.
Congregation:	God who is the greatest among us?
Leader:	Not the man who believes that power is about control and domination. But whoever receives a child in my name receives me.
Congregation:	God, who is the greatest among us?
Leader:	Not the man that rules his household with violence and instills only fear. But whoever receives a child in my name receives me.
Congregation:	God, who is the greatest among us? Not the man who uses power to dominate and exploit women and children sexually, and spread HIV/AIDS.
All:	Make us like little children, Oh God, humble and compassionate; able to love and embrace without prejudice; able to take care and protect without expecting any reward or favor; able to forgive as you have taught us to do. Amen

Suggested Symbols/ideas: Male Condoms, Bishops mitar, Slogans such as 'Real men don't rape – Real men practice safer sex', money notes, titles such as Manager, Director, etc.

By Cheryl Dibeela

7. Women

WOMEN'S SERVICE
Sermon Text: Proverbs 31:10-31

Introduction

The status of women in contemporary African societies has generated a lot of debate. Some activists maintain that women are oppressed by patriarchy, while others consider gender equity a foreign ideology. However, it is clear that married women are particularly vulnerable to HIV infection. Thus, what it means to be a virtuous woman requires radical interpretation in the light of the number of women infected by their husbands.

Despite being at the receiving end of the HIV/AIDS pandemic, women have done a sterling job in providing care. Many wives have nursed their husbands, sons, daughters and relatives often neglecting their own health. It is important that a new theology that does not offer women as sacrificial victims be developed. In the era of HIV/AIDS, married women need to be empowered to protect themselves. They are made on God's image. They should not surrender their lives in order to be deemed good wives. Factors such as culture and religion, lack of education and economic dependence have increased the vulnerability of women to HIV/AIDS. This oppressive structures need to be revisited and marriage needs to be re-conceptualized as partnership.

We Listen to the Word of God

The passage is a celebration of the good wife. It highlights the value of married women, outlining their centrality to the well-being of the household. Through devotion to her husband and accomplishing her chores, the good wife is an asset to her family and society. Being far more precious than jewels, a good wife appears to be measured by the amount of work that she accomplishes, rather than for her intrinsic value. It is important that this text be re-read because of its patriarchal influences.

We Apply the Word of God to Ourselves

WHAT CAN WE LEARN?
- Married women play a key role in their families;
- Cultural factors may force women to sacrifice themselves;
- Numerous tasks undertaken by housewives are often ignored;
- House-wives are exhausted, they need help from their husbands.

WHAT DO WE HAVE TO CONFESS?
- Exposing married women to HIV/AIDS;
- Refusing to recognize work done by women;
- Abandoning care of those affected by HIV/AIDS to women;
- That as men and husbands, we often neglect housework.

WHAT CAN WE THANKFUL FOR?
- Women provide care for the infected;
- Mothers continue to work for their families amidst poverty, pain and oppression;
- Most wives have remained faithful despite their husband's promiscuity;
- That men can make a difference in the spread of HIV/AIDS through faithfulness.

WHAT CAN WE PRAY FOR?
- Husbands should be sensitive and appreciate their wives;
- Family members, especially men, should participate in giving care in situations of HIV/AIDS;
- Wives should be empowered to protect themselves against HIV infection.

We Apply the Word of God to the Congregation

Let married women in the congregation discuss the following questions:
- Do they feel that their husbands and families appreciate their efforts?
- What should their families do to improve the situation?
- Do they get support when they provide care in HIV/AIDS contexts?
- Do husbands participate in the many chores of their homes?

Conclusion: A Word on Society

Society needs to overhaul its theory that women are long-suffers. Despite progress that has been made in raising awareness of gender issues in Africa, married women continue to suffocate, particularly in this era of HIV/AIDS. Cultural, religious, economic and other factors that increase the vulnerability of women should be overcome. The church must take a lead to empower women, for we were all created in God's image.

Song

Vana Mai,
Tiri masoja,
Ekudenga,
Tiri masoja aMwari,
Kana Satani akauya,
Tinomudhuura nebhaibheri.

Dear mothers,
We are soldiers of heaven,
We are God's soldiers,
If the devil (disease, pain, etc.) comes,
We will shoot it with the Bible.

(Popular chorus by women)
OR

Sweet Mother

Prayer of Confession by Men

God Almighty,
We thank you for the gift of women,
We praise you for their industry, tenderness and care,
We give you glory, God most high!
Forgive us, Lord, when we exploit women labor and love,
Forgive the times when we selfishly expose them to diseases.
Forgive us, Lord, when we take them for granted.
Strengthen us to acknowledge their humanity.
Help us to banish gender inequalities and violence.
We have gone wrong, gone astray.
By trivializing the status of women;
By not counting women's activities as valuable work;
By leaving all care for the sick to women;
By leaving all housework to our wives.
Living God, hear our prayers,
Through Jesus Christ. Amen

Poem: Daughters of Ethiopia

Groaning in faith,
Rejoicing in hope,
Effaced from official statistics,
Written in the Book of Life.

Feeding the hungry,
Comforting the lonely,
Nursing the sick,
Loving the outcasts.

Victims of patriarchy and vicious systems,
Bearing eloquent scars of torture,
Used and discarded,
Brutalized and squeezed.

Your spirit is unbroken,
The Spirit urges you on,
Daughters of Ethiopia,
We salute your courage and tenacity,
May the Lord of Justice and Mercy,
Reward your efforts a hundred fold!

Reject choking systems,
Overthrow stifling ideologies,
Embrace liberation,
Cherish freedom,
Daughters of faith,
YOUR HOUR HAS COME!!

Suggested objects: Carving of mother with child at her back, carrying firewood; white cloth; water, pictures of working women and men sitting under a tree, etc.

By Ezra Chitando

WOMEN'S SERVICE
Sermon Text: Ruth 1-2

This sermon can also be used as a sermon for widows.

Leader: Women of God, why are you here?
All: We gather in the name of the Creator God, as women of God who want to transform this world to one where there is justice for all. We call upon the Spirit of God to give us courage to effect the necessary change, and to unite us so that we speak with one voice. We pledge each other to work in solidarity to achieve our goal.

Greeting Song (Chichewa)
As they sing this song, they should greet each other.

LEADER: Inu anzathu // (Our Friends)
ALL: Sitinadziwe kuti tidzaonana // (We did not know that we will meet)
                 Moni Mulungu adalitse // (Greetings, God bless you)
                                      (2x)
Leader: Inu anzathu // (Our friends)
All: Moni // (Greetings) (3x)
                 Mulungu adalitse // (God bless you)
                       (Malawian Community Song)

Introduction

The position of women in the church and society varies from one church to another and from one culture to another. The dominant belief is that women are inferior to men, and women must always submit. Women are also denied leadership on the basis that a woman cannot lead men, only other women and children. It is for these reasons that women are treated like perpetual minors. The dangerous part is that women themselves have internalized their oppression and accepted it as coming from God. Therefore, in some cases, women oppress other women and oppose the women who seek the liberation of other women.

In spite of this, the existence of Churchwomen organizations in Africa is a symbol of solidarity among women. These organizations need to transform, so that they can become a mouthpiece on women's issues in the church and society. This is particularly urgent in this era of HIV/AIDS. The subordination of women to men puts women at high risk for HIV because it means that women do not have the power or right to negotiate for safer sex. Some of the issues that put women in the HIV/AIDS high risk category include: lack of education, economic dependence, cultural and religious teachings.

We Listen to the Word of God

Naomi, Ruth and Opah were widows. Ruth and Naomi formed a partnership for survival without the help of a man. They were proactive.

They made a journey from Moab to Bethlehem. It was a strategic journey for economic empowerment. Naomi had heard that the famine was over in Bethlehem. They returned at the time of harvesting wheat, the staple food of those people.

By God's providence, Ruth worked in the field of Boaz, a distant relative of Naomi's husband. Boaz showed kindness to Ruth, because Ruth had been kind to Naomi. Ruth is warned to remain in Boaz' field for fear of being abused by workers from other fields.

Ruth, encouraged by Naomi, initiated marriage to Boaz. They used patriarchal methods to actively change their situation. They subverted the system. Was Naomi using Ruth for her own ends? No, because Naomi told Ruth to go back and Ruth followed out of her free will. This is an example that women can be in solidarity with each other. Their solidarity was for survival. The age gap between them was not a barrier.

We Apply the Word of God to Ourselves

WHAT CAN WE LEARN FROM THE THREE WIDOWS?
- The majority of widows live in economic hardships in patriarchal societies;
- That powerless people can change their situation if they work together;
- When people are in economic desperation, they can end up in prostitution or being tricksters, not because they are inherently evil, but because of circumstances;
- Widows are also in danger of being sexually harassed by men since they do not have male protection, thereby are at risk of being infected by HIV;
- The strategy that Ruth used for economic survival could have lead Ruth to death if Boaz was HIV positive;
- It is difficult for older widows to remarry, as widowers tend to want to marry virgins not widows;
- We realize that Boaz responded respectfully to the needs of Ruth.

WHAT DO WE HAVE TO CONFESS?
- Have we given support to widows?
- Has the church taken a prophetic stand towards the dispossession of HIV/AIDS widows?
- Have we protected widows from sexual harassment?
- Have we empowered the women church groups to be supportive of the liberation of women?
- Have we given women space to be empowered economically, socially, sexually, theologically and economically?
- Have we promoted friendship and solidarity among women?

WHAT CAN WE BE THANKFUL FOR?
- That woman can survive after the death of their husbands and sons;
- God is on the side of widows;

- The church is commanded by God to take care of widows;
- Surviving male relatives can behave responsibility.

WHAT CAN WE PRAY FOR?
- Neglected, dispossessed and psychologically harassed widows who are not being looked after by anyone;
- The church to look after widows;
- Churchwomen groups to take seriously the issue of helping widows;
- God to give us courage to deal with women's issues in the church;
- God to continue to strengthen women as they look after their sick husbands and children, especially in the time of HIV/AIDS;
- Encourage dying spouses to write their wills.

We Apply the Word of God to the Congregation

WHAT CAN WE FEEL?
- Repentant for not taking care of widows and for not supporting women's cause for solidarity in the church;
- Encouraged by the formation of widows associations and women's groups that seek change for themselves.

WHAT CAN WE BE?
- A supportive community to the needs of widows and women groups.

WHAT CAN WE DO?
- Sponsoring widows for income generating projects;
- Promoting the formation of widows associations in our churches, so that we create space for widows to encourage each other;
- Show interest in the well-being of widows and their children;
- Actively oppose cultural practices that hinder the remarriage of widows;
- Actively oppose cultural practices that deny widows from inheriting their husbands' property;
- Actively oppose government rules that make widows as perpetual minors to their sons;
- Promote the writing of wills for all church members, so as to protect women from relatives that grab property after the death of husbands.

Conclusion: A Word on Society

There are many women in our societies who are going through similar situations to Naomi and Ruth. Women take care of their husbands who have AIDS until they die. But when they get sick, there is no one to take care of them. Sometimes when the woman is the first to get sick from AIDS, the husband will send her back to her people for care. In cases when the husband gets sick first, the wife is there for him up to the end. Such practices need to be challenged, so that both husband and wife take care of each other both in sickness and in health. The church needs to campaign for the legal protection of widows, especially over the issues of inheritance laws. There is need for a change of laws, even in the church about widows. The churches need to revisit their views about single mothers, widows and remarriage.

Song (Chichewa)

(*Chorus*)
Jehova, Jehova Atamandike // (Jehovah, Jehovah, should be praised)
Palipenso wina Mulungu // (There is no other God)
Ndimodzi yekha Jehova // (There is One Jehovah) (2x)

Iye ndiye Alepha // (He/she is Alpha)
Iye ndiye Omega // (He/she is Omega)
Oyamba ndi otsiliza // (The beginning and the end)
Palibenso wina Mulungu // (There is no other God)
Ndimodzi yekha, Jehova // (There is one Jehovah)
(*Repeat chorus*)

(A Malawian Community Song)

Prayer

Leader: Lord, we thank you because you are a faithful friend, a friend who sticks closer than a relative.

All: Lord, we thank you for a Christian community. Thank you for your call that we should take care of our widows. We accept our responsibility, Lord.

Leader: We commit the widows to you. Our prayer for them is that they may feel your presence in their lives and learn to lean on you as they walk through the journey of life. Help them to know that you are the husband of the widows and the father of the fatherless

All: We accept the challenge to change our church and cultural laws that have contributed to the abuse of widows. Have mercy on us Lord and give us the courage to transform our communities, to make them widow and women friendly. In Jesus' name, Amen

Symbols/object/ideas: Testimonies from widows, film from Zimbabwe on inheritance, scented candles, black dress, a bundle of wheat, musical instruments, etc.

By Isabel Apawo Phiri

8. Widows and Widowhood

SERVICE FOR WIDOWS
Sermon Text: Luke 18:1-8

Introduction

In the HIV/AIDS era, the plight and proliferation of widows has come to the fore. Married women lose husbands and become widows. In some African cultures they are expected to choose another husband within the siblings of their husbands. In other cases they are dispossessed of both their property and children. Sometimes they are accused of witchcraft, of having killed their husbands or having infected them with HIV/AIDS. Sometimes they are left poor by the disease itself, but also because they may be without work, skills or property, so they turn to sex work to survive. In many cultures they are subjugated to severe rituals of cleansing, since their bodies are held to be unclean. Most of the above experiences are not helpful in the area of HIV/AIDS prevention and provision of quality care. Further, their experiences are closely linked to gender inequalities that characterize most marriages, property ownership, stereotypes on origins of evil and stigmatization of women's bodies as unclean.

The Bible, both the Hebrew Bible and the New Testament, highlights the situation of widows on several occasions (Tamar, Ruth, Naomi and Opah). The prophets also highlight the plight of widows, depicting God as taking their side. Similarly, in the New Testament, Jesus makes several references to widows. Some examples include; raising up the son of a widow from death; the widow who gave the best; and the widow who followed the judge repeatedly, searching for justice. The latter constitutes the focus of this sermon, as the preacher/Bible study leader seeks to bring the congregation and society to be more sensitive to the plight and situation of widows in the HIV/AIDS era. This service seeks to highlight the plight of widows; to hear their needs in the area of HIV/AIDS prevention, provision of care, mitigation of impact, legal and spiritual guidance.

Story
Bring a widow to tell her story of struggle and survival.

We Listen to the Word of God

Reading of the Word (Luke 18:1-8)
DETAILS OF THE TEXT
Verse 1-2:
➤ The story is told to illustrate persistent prayer and persistent action. In the second verse, both setting (in a certain city) of the story and one of the characters (the judge) are introduced.

➤ Note that the setting is neutral, thus lending itself to universal application. That is, it was in a certain city—it could be any city: your city and my city where such characters are found. The preacher/Bible study leader should thus ask the congregation/participants if such characters exist in their city.

➤ Note that verse 2 explicates the character of the judge: "He neither feared God nor had respect for people." This is telling; how will he serve people or God if he has no respect for either?

Verse 3:
➤ The setting is re-iterated and another character of the story is introduced: "In that city there was a widow." First, define a widow culturally, economically and spiritually. Second, put it to the congregation/participants to see if widows exist in their city, and if widows are also seeking justice.

➤ The situation of the widow brings her to this judge, who respects no one. Note that she "Kept coming to the judge," this denotes persistence, but it may also denote desperation. It also underlines the negligence of the judge.

➤ "Grant me justice against my opponent," says the persistent widow to the judge. Why was she seeking justice? What kind of justice was she seeking? Who was her opponent? The text does not say. However, she was a widow. As a preacher/bible study leader, highlight the various injustices that confront widows and their many opponents. For example, this widow may have been dispossessed of her husband's property, her home, her children. The widow may have been accused of witchcraft and driven out of her home. Her opponents may very well be the relatives of her husband, her neighbors, culture and the legal system that does not protect her.

Verse 4-5:
➤ Highlight that the judge who has no fear for God or respect for people, ignores her. Public leaders and workers, who are serving people, can hardly serve if they do not fear God or respect people.

➤ Ask the congregation/participants if such civil servants exist in the church and in their country. Ask if they can be described in such terms, if they have ever had such attitude and how it affected those who seek help from them.

➤ The persistence of the desperate widow, however, gets to the judge. He grants her justice, but for wrong reasons, "So that she may not wear me out by continually coming." He serves her not because he believes she deserves justice, but to get rid of her.

Verses 6-7:
➤ Jesus now gives his interpretation and opinion on such a judge.

➤ Verse 6 Jesus says, "Listen to what the unjust judge says." Two points are notable here. First, Jesus says, "Listen" the verb calls our attention denoting emphasis, surprise, disgust and protest. Second, Jesus calls him "the unjust judge." Why is his behaviour unacceptable and unjust? This is stated in verse seven.

➤ In verse 7, Jesus asks, "And will not God grant justice to the chosen ones who cry to God day and night?" This is a rhetorical question that clearly expects a positive answer. That is, yes, God will grant justice to widows and to all who cry to God day and night! Several points should be highlighted by the preacher/Bible study leader from this verse. First, the fact that Jesus expressed himself in a question is notable. It is emphasis. The fact that Jesus refers to God as a God who grants justice. God is a fair judge, a God of justice. Underline the fact that Jesus counts this widow among the chosen ones who call upon God day and night.

➤ Emphasis that the poor, the underprivileged, the marginalized, the oppressed, including widows—are God's chosen ones. God listens to their search for justice.

➤ "Will God delay long in helping them?" Jesus asks, thus underlining that it was, and still is unacceptable for all those who are in power to deny, or to delay justice to widows and all the marginalized. The point is clear here: justice delayed, is justice denied!

Verse 8:
➤ "I tell you, God will quickly grant justice to them," Jesus says. God is a just God, a fair judge, a judge who delivers justice in time and to all those who need it, especially the widows and all other marginalized people. God's justice is timely—it is quickly delivered. The preacher/Bible study leader must underline that this means that God does not allow oppression or expect the church to be tolerant of it.

➤ Underline that the justice of God to widows and all the oppressed, underline God's attentiveness and service must mean that in all our cities we do not have any right to deny the rights of widows. They must be quickly met.

➤ In sum, the preacher/Bible study leader must bring it to the attention of the congregation/participants that this passage is comparative. It compares the just God and the unjust judge. In so doing, it seeks to underline in no uncertain terms that if God is a just God, who acts promptly, then none of us and no city of the world should wait too long before it grants widows and all other oppressed people, who cry to God day and night, their justice. Second, the meaning of the points of this story must be grasped in the tone of the story.

We Apply the Word of God to Ourselves

WHAT CAN WE LEARN?
• That we fail God whenever we entertain oppression;
• That justice delayed is justice denied;
• That God cares for the marginalized and expects us to care;
• That in many cities there are desperate widows and powerful people who neglect their duties.

WHAT DO WE HAVE TO CONFESS?
• That many times we have played the unjust judge;
• We have not listened to the cries of our widows;
• We have not set up services to meet the needs of widows;
• We have not been advocates for the needs of widows.

WHAT CAN WE BE THANFUL FOR?
- For a God who cares, listens, and who is just to all widows;
- For the families that have protected their widows;
- For assertive and persistent widows, who seek their justice;
- For children who have supported their widowed mothers;
- For NGOs that work with and for the needs of widows.

WHAT CAN WE PRAY FOR?
- For the protection of vulnerable widows;
- For a church, government and NGOs that are supportive;
- For promotion of cultures that protects widows.

We Apply the Word of God to the Congregation

WHAT CAN WE FEEL?
- Compassion for widows.

WHAT CAN WE BE?
- A listening church and society;
- A justice granting church to widows and all the marginalized.

WHAT CAN WE DO?
- Set up legal and counseling services for dispossessed widows;
- Set up day care centers for HIV/AIDS positive widows;
- Carry out home-based care for sick and bedded widows;
- Work with NGOs that serve widows;
- Assume public advocacy for unjustly treated widows;
- Fight gender injustice which denies widows their rights.

Conclusion: A Word on Society

While groups such as children, PLWAs, grandmothers, and women are identified for how they are affected by HIV/AIDS, it is rare to find services that target the needs of widows. One sometimes gets the feeling that if a husband dies of HIV/AIDS then the wife will quickly follow. This need not be the case. This silence can also reflect the cultural position of the widows as powerless people. It is imperative for the church to highlight their situation in the society and to champion their rights.

Suggested Song/Poem

Night has Fallen
(Thuma Mina, No. 208)

Or any hymn of your choice.

199

Closing Prayer

Leader: Like Ruth, let us pray and pledge our full support to all widows:

All: "Do not press me to leave you or to turn back from following you
Where you go, I will go, where you lodge, I will lodge,
Your people shall be my people and your God my God.

Where you die, I will die and there I will be buried
May the Lord do thus and so to me
And more as well until death parts us." Amen (Ruth 1:16-17)

Suggested Symbols/ideas: A picture of a widow, a story of a widow, black clothes, or any other symbols that captures mourning within your particular context and church background, etc.

By Musa W. Dube

SERVIÇO PARA VIÙVAS
Texto sugerido: Ruth 1:1-22

Introdução

Em África existem muitas mulheres. Entre elas encontramos vários grupos: Mães solteiras, abandonadas, divorciadas, viúvas,etc. Este grupo de senhoras vive marginalizado. São vistas como imorais, feiticeiras, ladras dos maridos das outras, propagadoras do HIV/SIDA. A Bíblia fala-nos de três mulheres pobres tanto em bens materiais como em relações humanas. Ao contrário daquilo que muitas vezes acontece, essas mulheres uniram-se na luta pela sobrevivência e pelo direito à vida e à família. Naomi, é um exemplo raro de uma sogra que ama as suas noras e deseja-lhes o bem. As duas noras são também exemplo raro de dedicação às pessoas de idade avançada.O HIV/SIDA é uma doença que desafia os lares para uma união efectiva e duradoira.

Escutemos a Palavra de Deus

Leia o texto. Sublinhe com um lápis as palavras mais importantes.
DETALHES
VV 1-2:
➢ Falam da fome e de como ela provoca deslocação de famílias à busca de melhor sorte.

VV. 3-5:
➢ Mostram como desgraças sucessivas abateram aquela família. Mostram também o seu desgosto provocado pela falta de descendência.

VV. 6-14:
➢ Relatam-nos o quanto as tres mulheres se amavam mas que apesar disso tinham que se separar. Finalmente uma delas decidiu regressar à casa da sua mãe.

VV. 15-18:
➢ São uma verdadeira escola de amor e de fé.

VV. 19-22:
➢ Falam-nos do regresso de Naomi com a sua nora à Belém e de como foram recebidas.

A Palavra de Deus para nós

QUE PODEMOS APRENDER?
- Que a fome criou e continua a criar deslocação de pessoas e animais de um lado para o outro.
- Que a morte de ente queridos, muitas vezes cria problemas difíceis de ultrapassar.
- O texto deixa bem claro que só o amor entre as pessoas enlutadas pode ajudar a encontrar soluções para os problemas que se levantam.
- Na era do HIV/SIDA as famílias devem unir-se para ajudar uns aos outros.

QUE TEMOS DE CONFESSAR?
- Que nos nossos lares não há harmonia principalmente entre sogras e noras.
- Que apesar de sermos crentes, temos dificuldade de aceitar a morte de pessoas que amamos.
- Que muitas vezes as viúvas são expulsas e arrancadas os seus bens depois da morte dos seus maridos.

QUE DEVEMOS PEDIR NAS NOSSAS ORAÇÕES?
- Que Deus nos perdoe pela falta de amor para com os nossos semelhantes.
- Que as mulheres deixem de acusar umas às outras quando surge uma morte.
- Pelo fim de hostilidades que provocam deslocações.

A Palavra de Deus para a sociedade

- Que sentimentos tiveram depois da leitura do texto?
- que aprenderam sobre relacções humanas?
- Que pensam sobre a atitude de Naomi?
- Que pensam sobre a atitude das suas noras?
- Que faria você numa situação idêntica?

Oração
Deus de amor e de compaixão, aproximamo-nos de ti, cheios (as) de pesar, por constantemente ignorar-mos os teus mandamentos cheios de sabedoria. Por actos e palavras pecamos contra ti. Quando as desgraças batem à porta da nossa casa, esquecemos de imediato que nos amas, e começamos com acusações mútuas. Proteja-nos Senhor, do pecado e da morte. Ressuscite em nós, a bondade, a esperança e o amor, em nome de Jesus Cristo. Amen

Canção
Escolhe uma canção que esteja de acordo com o sermão.

Objectos: Uma fotografia representando uma mulher enlutada, ou um casamento, ou um funeral, etc.

Por: Felicidade N. Cherinda

9. HOMOSEXUALS

Suggested Sermon Text: I John 4:7-21

Call to Worship

Leader 1:	You are God the Creator, You created all of us in your image.
All:	In your Garden there are many different flowers, And you created all of them good.
Leader 2:	You are God the Creator, You created life in wide diversities.
All:	In your universe there are billions of shinning stars, And you created all of them good.
Leader 3:	You are the Creator God, You created us black, white, yellow, tall, short, men and women.
All:	In your world there are many languages and ethnic groups, And you created all of them good.
Leader 4:	You are the Creator God, You created us with a range of sexual orientations.
All:	We are a beautiful rainbow people, And you created all of us good.

Introduction

The identity of homosexuality is perhaps one of the most difficult and least understood identities for the African church in general. Many church leaders reject homosexuality outright, together with those who carry this identity. As a result, homosexuals are rarely out with their status in most African churches and societies. The fact that HIV/AIDS was first discovered amongst the gay community was interpreted by some church leaders as God's punishment. The reality of HIV/AIDS is otherwise, as the infection is now largely transmitted through heterosexuals, especially in Africa. Despite the African churches' rejection of homosexuality, it is certainly a reality amongst African people since some languages have a name for it, indicating that is was always known.

In the HIV/AIDS era, the discrimination of homosexuals means they are often deprived of services that pertain to prevention and provision of quality care. This discrimination means that some homosexuals are forced to hide their identity, to marry wives and then to live with a double sexual life; a secret one and a publicly accepted one. In addition, since homosexuality is not openly talked about in most African societies and churches, emerging research indicates that some youngsters are opting for homosexual sex, believing that one would not get HIV/AIDS from it. In short, the discrimination of homosexuals and the silence that surrounds it does not only expose them to HIV/AIDS infection and lack of quality care, it affects all of us—even heterosexuals, for we are a community.

Does biblical theology give us room to accept and love those who are different from us? Does it call us to welcome strangers—those whom we do not know and understand? It would seem yes. Even those church members who are strongly convinced that their faith allows no room for homosexuality must still remember that the Bible counsels us strongly against judging and self-righteousness (Luke 6: 41-42; Luke 18:9-14; Matthew). It counsels us to love and calls us to inclusive fellowship (Luke 5:29-32; 15:1-2). We are urged to leave all judgment to God (Romans 12:19-20). But we do have a role to play; namely, to love our neighbors (John 14: 34-35; Mark 12: 28-34; Matthews 22: 38-40; Romans 13:8-10). The commandment to love each fellow human being was given to the church. Given that our faith and baptism in Christ, makes us one (Galatians 3:26-28), it is underlined that, "Those who say, "I love God," and hate their sisters and brothers are lairs; for those who do not love a brother or a sister whom they have seen, cannot love God whom they have not seen" (I John 4:20).

Song
Amazing Grace, How Sweet the Sound

Reading the Text: I John 4:7-21

We Listen to the Word of God

DETAILS OF THE TEXT
Verse 7-8:
> - "Let us love one another," the writer encourages those who are in the Christian fellowship to share or give love to each other. Note the reasons that the author gives: a) "Because love is from God," and b) Everyone who loves is born of God and knows God." The act of loving is an attestation that we have the Spirit of God.

> - Note and underline that verse 8 emphasizes verse 7; namely, "Whoever does not love does not know God, for God is Love." In short, it cannot be that we call ourselves Christians or a people of God if we do not love. The moment we fail to love—regardless of what reason we give—then we have failed to reflect the nature of God. We are ignorant people—we lack the knowledge of who God is.

> - "God is Love"; the text identifies God with love. We express our knowledge and relationship with God, our capacity to love: to love ourselves, to love our families, neighbors and the strangers—those who are different from us, be it racially, ethnically, gender wise, economically, culturally or by sexual orientation.

Verse 9-10:
> - God's love for us was manifested in God's act of giving, of loving us first, before we loved God. Love is about giving; and giving something precious. But all of us were given love by God, "Not that we loved God, but God loved us." It was unconditional. It was a free gift. We know God if we are capable of loving those who are unlike us, those who are different- and being to love them unconditionally.

Verses 11-12:

➤ The author underlines, "Beloved, since God loved us so much, we also ought to love one another." Those who have received love must give love.

➤ How do we measure that we are a godly people? Verse 12 says, "If we love one another, God lives in us and God's love is perfected in us."

Verses 13-15:

➤ God's Spirit was given to us, and we know that God abides in us, and we abide in God, through our capacity to love one another.

➤ Further, this Spirit of God enables us to, "Confess that Jesus is the Son of God."

➤ Underline that people in our fellowship, or even those who are outside, should not judged to be ungodly or unchristian because they are different from us. Rather, we should ask if they are capable of loving and confessing Jesus. These are the Christian attestations that the Spirit of God abides in them, that they abide in God, and God abides in them.

Verses 16-19:

➤ These verses underline what has been said above; namely that, "God is love, and those who abide in love, abide in God, and God abides in them."

➤ Note that the text speaks of fear, "There is no fear in love, but perfect love casts out fear" (v. 18). Often, fear gets on the way of love, especially when we meet those who are different, those who are not like us—denominationally, nationally, religiously, racially, culturally, ethnically, sexually, in gender and economically. What is different is unknown, hence sometimes brews fear, for it threatens our reality with another reality. This response to difference is unfortunate and ungodly, for God is the author of diversity and the author of love. If we know God as the creator of all, then we will not fear difference, but love, for God is love.

➤ The author repeats (and repetition is emphasis in biblical literature); "We love because God first loved us" (v. 19). This was a free gift to all of us, and we should give it out too.

Verses 20-21:

➤ Highlight and underline to the listeners, that verses 20-21 are not only the summary of what has been said, but perhaps, one of the most beautiful texts of Christian faith—one whose potential is yet to be fully realized.

➤ First, the text empathically states that those who say 'I love God,' and hate their brothers and sisters are liars. Put it to the congregation, ask them if they hate someone or a certain group of people? Underline that according to this text we cannot reconcile loving God and hating some people. If we hate people, we only delude ourselves if we think we love God, we are 'liars.'

➤ Second, the text gives a strong reason, "For those who do not love a brother or sister whom they have seen, cannot love God whom they have not seen."

> The importance of these verses is in underlining that our Christian spiritually is based on the capacity of being able to live and to relate respectfully with our neighbors and with all people. Peaceful relationships, respect for all, acknowledging the human dignity of all people, seeing the image of God in all people: these are imperatives. These are godly acts. If we are capable of these, then we have a relationship with God, we know God, we love God, we abide in God and God abides in us. The Spirit of God is in us, if we love. Words cannot express what a healed and wonderful world we can have and how many lives would be saved from violence and war, if we knew and practiced just this: *Loving one another!*

We Apply the Word of God to Ourselves

WHAT CAN WE LEARN?
- That God is love;
- That we are commanded to love one another;
- That God loved us unconditionally and still loves us;
- That loving God begins with loving those whom we see.

WHAT DO WE HAVE TO CONFESS?
- We do not love all people unconditionally;
- We are often hindered to love, by judging others and by fear of differences;
- Our attitudes towards different sexual identities, genders, ethnic backgrounds, class and age hinder us from loving;
- We confess that our lack of love caused many wars, deaths of millions, hindered HIV/AIDS prevention and exposed those that we marginalize, especially homosexuals.

WHAT CAN WE BE THANKFUL FOR?
- That God loves and calls us to love unconditionally;
- That through faith and baptism, we are one in Christ; (Galatians 3:26-28)
- We have the opportunity to repent and to start loving others;
- Our fellowship and society has given us opportunity to know and to appreciate those who are different from us as worthy, and God fearing like us, or even better than us; (Luke 10:25-37)
- That, as African people, we have witnessed the struggle for black people and for women, who were discriminated against for their differences and we have learned from these to resist ethnic and sexually based discrimination;
- That God is the creator of diversity.

WHAT CAN WE PRAY FOR?
- For commitment to love and give justice to all people;
- For a church that is an example of unconditional love.

We Apply the Word of God to the Congregation

WHAT CAN WE BE?
- An inclusive and loving community;
- A safe home for all people who are rejected by larger society.

WHAT CAN WE DO?
- Set up support groups for gay people in our churches;
- Allow gay people to come out with their status;
- Supportively work with NGOs that focus on gay people.

Conclusion: A Word on Society

One of the amazing observations about society is that while God created diversity and created us all in God's image and God's likeness, we have hardly embraced and celebrated these differences, nor realized the dignity of each person and of creation as a whole. As people, we deem ourselves worthy of rejecting that which God has created and blessed. We fear and hate the 'other'. Thus wars of hate based of ethnicity, race, gender, nationality and religion have plagued our world. The greatest tragedy, however, is that we have never learned from these wars of hate to avoid violence, to begin to love and to accept each other. One war follows another. Millions have died and millions are still dying. Wars remain on the drawing boards of many leaders—the first and two thirds world alike. People who have themselves been victims of racism, anti-Semitism, ethnic cleansing, gender oppression, etc. quite easily forget their experiences and struggles for humanity, and become oppressors of other groups on the basis of their differences. The discrimination of homosexuals is one such example, one that we need to tackle, particularly in the HIV/AIDS struggle.

Song
Oh Lord my God when I in Awesome Wonder.

Closing Prayer
Leader:
Creator God, we have sinned against your creation,
When we discriminate people on the basis of their color, gender, ethnicity,
Class, health and sexual orientation. This discrimination has exposed these
Groups to HIV/AIDS infection and lack of quality care. We have been
Hypocritical, for we have failed to love others, while we claim to love you.
All: Forgive us Lord and teach us how to love one another.

Exchanging Peace

Turn to each of your neighbors, hold their hands in your hands, look them in the eye and say, "I love you with the love of God, for I can see in you the glory of God."

Objects/symbols: Rainbow drawing, bouquet of mixed flowers beautifully arranged; abstract of carving of two figures holding hands, a purple cloth or any other idea or symbol that may be appropriate for your context and audience.   By Musa W. Dube

10. People Living with HIV/AIDS

People Living With HIV/AIDS (PLWHA)
Sermon Text: Jeremiah 17:5-10

Instructions: Get the youth group to dramatize the stigma experienced by PLWHA, or get a PLWHA to share his/her experiences. Even better, invite a PLWHA society to church and let them talk about what they do, as well as their experiences.

Introduction

HIV/AIDS has affected sub-Saharan Africa severely. It is the leading cause of death, as well as being an epidemic within other social epidemics. Its impact has been greatest among the most vulnerable groups, such as the poor, displaced persons, prisoners, women and children. Despite progress in research, many PLWHA in Africa do not receive adequate health care due to factors such as accessibility and affordability of drugs, but also due to HIV/AIDS stigma and discrimination.

Although the church has been active in providing care for PLWHA, it has also been responsible for some of the stigma. The tendency to associate HIV/AIDS with promiscuity and immorality, or to see it as a form of divine judgment has increased stigma. Consequently, the church has not become the alternative space where PLWHA can feel welcome. The church has also not raised its prophetic voice as part of its advocacy work. Access to information, prevention and care are contemporary challenges, and the church should play a meaningful role in this regard.

We Listen to the Word of God

The passage emphasizes the need to trust in the Lord. As opposed to arrogance and a false sense of self-sufficiency, the church should be a trusting community. Even when HIV/AIDS threatens a sense of the future, the church should remain firm. When the heat of HIV/AIDS and its attendant problems comes, the community of faith should not falter.

Encourage members to debate the meaning of the sentence; "God promises to give every person according to their ways, according to his doings". While some have used the sentence as evidence that PLWHA have received what they deserve, indicate that judgment is the sole prerogative of God. Also, highlight factors such as rape, parent to child transmission, marital infidelity and others methods of HIV infection. Many good people get infected by HIV/AIDS. We cannot simply equate HIV/AIDS with immorality.

We Apply the Word of God to Ourselves

WHAT CAN WE LEARN?
- We need to continue trusting in God despite the HIV/AIDS pandemic;
- Judgment should be left to God;
- PLWHAs can still lead fulfilling and useful lives.

WHAT DO WE HAVE TO CONFESS?
- Failing to overcome stigma faced by PLWHAs;
- Doubting God's love in the face of HIV/AIDS;
- Failure to make our churches PLWHA friendly.

WHAT CAN WE THANKFUL FOR?
- Some members of society, particularly women, have provided care for PLWHA.

WHAT CAN WE PRAY FOR?
- The church should play a leading role in fighting discrimination and other factors that fuel HIV infection;
- Individuals who actively support PLWHAs;
- The power to refrain from playing God and judging PLWHAs;
- Talking up advocacy against national and international corruption.

We Apply the Word of God to the Congregation

- How often have we sinned by usurping God's throne and pronouncing judgment on PLWHAs?
- What can members do to welcome PLWHAs to their places of worship?
- Do members still trust in God, even as they bury loved ones virtually everyday?

Conclusion: A Word on Society

PLWHAs face multiple struggles, and society could help by overcoming stigma. Leaders at the family, church, village, provincial, national and global levels, ought to actively support PLWHAs. The provision of quality care should also be pursued vigorously. Above all, factors that increase the spread of HIV/AIDS should be tackled urgently.

Song
We Have a Miracle Working God (CLG Hymn Book, No. 135)
OR

Murapi ari pano
Chiremba wekudenga
Auya pasi pano
Kurapa mwoyo yedu
(Community song)

Prayer

Almighty God, Healer of Healers,
We come before your throne of mercy.
You sent your son and he bore our iniquities.
We pray that your Spirit lighten our hearts.
Touch us in your special way.
Unto us whisper words of healing and comfort.
Into our hearts pour the spirit of trust.
Transform us to become like the tree planted by water.
Lord, we know you have plans for us,
Plans for good and not for evil.
When our bodies hurt.
When our spirits are low.
When our anxieties wear us down.
We pray for endurance and hope.
Dear God, we know you listen to our prayers.
Your Spirit intercedes on our behalf.
Through our Lord and Savior, Jesus Christ we pray. Amen

Poem
TRUST IN THE LORD

Aches, aches, aches,
Searing pain,
Soaring doubt,
Deepening despair,

My children!
These little ones, the ones you so love?
Should I leave them now, tender as they are?
Why do you hide your face, God of love?
Lord, let this cup pass!

As I sit alone in silence,
A still small voice reassures me,
In the Lord I take refuge,
For thou art with me,
Thy rod and thy staff,
They comfort me,

More than a conqueror,
Heir of the kingdom,
Bearer of the promise,
I shall trust in you forever.

Suggested objects/symbols/ideas: Red ribbons over the cross (solidarity); green plants (vitality), PLWHA, T-shirts with reminders, Logo of PLHWA, 2002 World AIDS Day Logo.

By Ezra Chitando

209

11. Community Leadership

Sermon Text: Nehemiah 1-4

Introduction

Community mobilization and leadership are essential and imperative for the Christians to address the problems related to HIV/AIDS in our countries. This involves a passion and concern for the sufferings experienced by people around us. It requires initiative and vision. As community leaders we ought to lead on behalf of God, rather than with our own interests. Leadership is not a 'one-person show', but it involves cooperate support. This is the kind of leadership that led Nehemiah to rebuild the city of Jerusalem.

We Listen to the Word of God

DETAILS OF THE TEXT
➤ Nehemiah heard of the situation in Jerusalem, and what he heard moved him into action. He did not respond because of his official appointment to the palace, or because of his connections by birth, but rather because he was concerned with the crisis that faced the people in Jerusalem.

➤ Nehemiah's grief and concern for his comrades in Jerusalem drove him into a prolonged period of fasting and prayer. Nehemiah wept bitterly over the state of affairs.

➤ Nehemiah involved the cooperation of others in his plans to rebuild the city of Jerusalem. He also approached the king for support. He encountered a lot of opposition in his plans to rebuild the walls, but because of his dependence on God, he is able to withstand them.

➤ Nehemiah does a thorough inspection of the city walls, and carefully formulates a plan of operation. After thorough preparation, he is able to spur everybody into action. In spite of increased opposition, Nehemiah's mobilization and good leadership brings forth victory for the people of Jerusalem.

We Apply the Word of God to Ourselves

WHAT CAN WE LEARN?
• That words without action mean nothing;
• That each of us has a contribution to make towards improving the conditions of HIV/AIDS.

WHAT DO WE HAVE TO CONFESS?
• That we do not make the first steps in providing leadership;
• That we are often too comfortable with our own lives (what we eat, our own health, etc) and do not get moved into improving the lives of others;

- That as the church leaders, community leaders, and family leaders, we have not sufficiently spoken out concerning HIV/AIDS prevention and care;
- That as church leaders we have not taken public leadership to fight stigma and discrimination;
- That as men, we have not yet made the differences in HIV/AIDS prevention through faithfulness to our partners, abstaining or practicing safer sex.

WHAT CAN WE BE THANKFUL FOR?
- For the many community activists who try and make a difference to people living with HIV/AIDS, the orphans due to HIV/AIDS, medical treatment, support groups, etc.;
- For the leaders in the country that take these issues as important and a big concern;
- For PLWHA's who are out with their HIV status, fighting stigma and discrimination;
- HIV/AIDS care givers.

WHAT CAN WE PRAY FOR?
- That we do not separate social action from our Christian commitment, and so always ask for God's continual guidance;
- For renewed vision and inspiration in our leadership;
- For fighting against death and protecting life.

We Apply the Word of God to our Church/Society

WHAT CAN WE DO?
- Do research on aspects affecting people, so that we might know what kind of needs are in our society;
- Arrange educational talks around HIV/AIDS;
- Do training on leadership, so as to equip people with the necessary skills.

Suggested idea

As leader, one could use cartoon characters or drawings to tell the story as it is set out in Nehemiah:
- The broken wall;
- Nehemiah's personal response to the crisis;
- Personal and Cooperative Prayer;
- Nehemiah's interview with the King;
- They face many adversaries;
- Nehemiah inspects the city wall;
- They rise up and build.

The leader could then follow a participatory approach by letting people draw their own broken walls with regard to HIV/AIDS in their societies. Let the members talk about these broken walls in groups. The following topics could be used for discussions:
- Let people unpack their individual responses to the broken walls: how do they feel - are they moved at all with emotions by what they see;
- Their cooperative initiatives: what can they do - have they done anything about

211

it so far – do they think they might want to do something about it;
- Their prayer response: does God know how they feel about these broken walls, have they confessed and interceded on behalf of the people;
- Who would be important to network with: what skills and influences are important for their mission.
- What opposition might they face?
- What action plan could they formulate?
- Are they fully equipped to raise up build those broken walls: where/how/when could they start?

Song
The leader may choose any appropriate song.

Prayer
Dear God, our builder, you have all the building materials needed to construct our societies. You have all the strength to put wisdom on all that has fallen apart in our lives. You have the wisdom to re shape our world. Inspire us with all your wisdom, strength and love, to rebuild the broken walls in our community. Amen

Suggested objects: Bricks, cement, tools for building, clothes used for building, pictures of concerns in society.

By Cheryl Dibeela

12. HIV/AIDS Workers

Suggested Reading: Matthew 9:35-38 and John 21:15-18

Introduction

It is internationally recognized that most HIV/AIDS workers (planners, activists, caregivers, programmers, educators, trainers, advocates, counselors, etc.) suffer burn out. There are several reasons for this. HIV/AIDS in itself is a huge field, one who undertakes HIV/AIDS work will inevitably get more than enough to do—everyday, all the 365 days of the year! It is an urgent work. It is critical. It is about saving lives, so its workers can hardly distance their bodies, souls and minds from this stressful urgency. It is also depressing work in the sense that one comes face to face with suffering and death (especially those who are in home-based care such as nurses and doctors) and one can easily lose hope, and the meaning of life.

It is almost always the case that there are insufficient workers in all fields of HIV/AIDS. The shortage is partly because it is a relatively new field. It is also because of the stigma—very few people want to identify themselves with HIV/AIDS work. Some still think it is a health issue. Some are just indifferent. Others are ignorant. It is also because while it is largely a voluntary service, it nonetheless demands all your time. The result is that those who have courageously come forward, have more work than they can handle. They suffer from burn out. They are often traveling (house to house, around the village, city, nation, internationally, etc). They are away from family and unable to take care of their own health. It is important that HIV/AIDS workers be recognized, to raise their morale, to strengthen them, but also to call for more people to stand and be counted. This service seeks to affirm those who work with HIV/AIDS, and be a call for more workers.

Call to Worship

Leader 1:   "How beautiful upon the mountains,
Are the feet of the messenger,
Who announces peace,
Who brings good news,
Who announces salvation,
Who says to Zion,
Your God reigns." (Isaiah 52:7)

HIV/AIDS Workers

Yet many times we are weary and totally exhausted by HIV/AIDS work,
for "The harvest is plentiful, but the laborers are few. Therefore ask the Lord of the harvest to send out laborers into the harvest." (Luke 10:2)

Song
Nkosi Sikelele iAfrica

Prayer by HIV/AIDS Workers

Loving and caring God, thank you, for you call us to love and serve your people.
You call us to be healing hands in your hurting world.
You send us to compassion, to suffer with those who suffer.
Day and night we labor to comfort your people.
Yet many times we are depressed by the amount of suffering we see.
And many times we are totally exhausted by the amount of work we have to do.
We often neglect our health and families in the HIV/AIDS struggle.
Help us, Lord. Lord, renew our strength. Amen

Song
Thuso // Help us help us (14x)
(© Thuso Tiego, from the album *Thuso, 2002*)

Leader 2:   "Those who wait for the Lord shall renew their strength,
They shall renew their strength,
They shall mount up with wings like eagles,
They shall run and not be weary,
They shall walk and not faint." (Isaiah 40:31)

Song

U Jesu maka bongwe // May Jesus be praised (4x)

Se hamba naye // We walk with Jesus
Si hlala naye // We sit with Jesus
Si lala naye // We sleep with Jesus
Sivuka naye // And wake up with him (2x)

U Jesu maka bongwe // May Jesus be praised (4x)
(Anonymous)

First Reading: Matthew 9:35-38

"Then Jesus went about all the cities and villages, teaching and proclaiming the good news of the kingdom, and curing every disease and every sickness. When he saw the crowds, he had compassion for them, because they were harassed and helpless like sheep without a shepherd. Then he said to his disciples, "The harvest is plentiful, but the laborers are few.""

Second Reading: John 21:15-18

When they had finished breakfast, Jesus said to Simon Peter, "Simon, son of John, do you love me more than these?" He said to him, "Yes, Lord; you know that I love you." Jesus said to him, "Feed my lambs." A second time he said to him, "Simon, son of John, do you love me?" He said to him, "Yes, Lord; you know that I love you." Jesus said to him, "Tend my sheep." He said to him the third time, "Simon son of John, do you love me?" Peter felt hurt because he said to him the third time, "Do you love me?" And he said to him, "Lord, you know everything; you know that I love you." Jesus said to him, "Feed my sheep."

Leader 3: "Then I heard the voice of the Lord saying,
Whom shall I send, and who will go for us?
All: Here am I; send me." (Isaiah 6:8)
"Until justice rolls down like waters
And righteousness like an ever-flowing stream." (Amos 5:24)
Send us Lord.
Testimony 1: A Home-based caregiver
The Rest:
Renew us, Lord. Renew our spirits and minds.
Help us to see your face in the face of the sick.

Leader hands a certificate/token of appreciation.

Testimony 2: A Grandmother caring for orphans
The Rest:
Renew us, Lord. Renew our spirits and minds.
Restore our physical strength and hope, oh Lord.

Leader hands a certificate/token of appreciation.

Testimony 3:   A child-headed family
The Rest:
Renew us, Lord. Renew our hope for the future.
Restore our faith in your unfailing care, guidance and presence.

Leader hands a certificate/token of appreciation.

Testimony 4:   HIV/AIDS Counselor or social worker
The Rest:
Renew us, Lord. Renew our service to your people.
Restore our commitment to comfort your people.

Leader hands a certificate/token of appreciation.

Testimony 5: Health care-givers (nurses and doctors)
The Rest:
Renew us, Lord. Renew our compassion for your suffering people.
Help us to see your image in each sick and suffering person.

Leader hands a certificate of appreciation.

Testimony 6:   A village HIV/AIDS educator
The Rest:
Renew us, Lord. Renew our dedication to people.
Restore our communities, fill us with joy and hope.

Leader hands a certificate/token of appreciation.

Testimony 7:   A national HIV/AIDS worker
The Rest:
Renew us Lord.   Renew our vision for a healed nation.
Restore our nation to its peace, rebuild it broken spirit.

Leader hands a certificate/token of appreciation.

Testimony 8:   An International HIV/AIDS activist
The Rest:
Renew us Lord. Renew and heal your creation.
Restore goodness to all members of the earth community.

Leader hands a certificate/token of appreciation.

Testimony 9: HIV/AIDS program person
The Rest:
Renew us Lord. Renew our energy and commitment
Restore our physical, mental and spiritual vigor to be healing hands

Leader hands a certificate/token of appreciation.

Testimony 10: A PLWHA activist
The Rest:
Renew us Lord. Renew our minds, spirits and society.
Restore and re-fill our bodies with your healing touch.

Leader hands a certificate/token of appreciation.

Testimony 11: A Youth HIV/AIDS activist
The Rest:
Renew us Lord. Renew our love and hope
Fill us again with your Spirit of Power and the Spirit of fire.

Leader hands a certificate/token of appreciation.

Song

U Jesu maka bongwe // May Jesus be praised (4x)
Se hamba naye // We walk with Jesus
Si hlala naye // We sit with Jesus
Si lala naye // We sleep with Jesus
Sivuka naye // And wake up with him (2x)

U Jesu maka bongwe // May Jesus be praised (4x)
(Anonymous)

Leader: "The harvest is plentiful, but the laborers are few, therefore, ask the Lord of harvest to send laborers into his harvest."

Song

Ke tla roma mang // Whom shall I send? (3x)
Roma mang ko lefatsheng // Shall I send to the world

Ntate roma nna // Send me Lord (3x)
Roma nna ko lefatsheng // Send me Lord to the world
(Anonymous)

Call to Serve
Those who have not been involved in HIV/AIDS work; who wish to start; or to contribute to both prevention and provision of care are, called to stand and come forward.

Prayer of Dedication
Creator God, in this HIV/AIDS era, the harvest is plentiful and the laborers are few. We thank you for the few laborers that are carrying heavy burdens. Renew their strength and energy to serve. Here, then are your people, more servants. They have heard you calling, "Whom shall I send, who shall go for me?" They have heard you say, "Who shall undertake HIV/AIDS prevention and provision of care to the sick for me?" They have heard you say, "The harvest is plentiful, but the laborers are few." They have come forward to you. They are saying, "Here we are, send us Lord."

We dedicate them to you and your care. Creator God, take their hands and feet and send them to every home and corner where they are needed. Take their hearts and minds and fill them with compassionate energy. Take their eyes and ears help them to see pain and to hear the cries of all who suffer as your pain and cry. Anoint them now and fill them with your Holy Spirit, your Spirit of power and fire. We thank you that you have already heard our prayers. Amen

Leader gives a pebble to each new person as a reminder for their pledge to God and their dedication to serve in the HIV/AIDS struggle.

Commissioning

Go with the God of compassion.
Go with Emmanuel, the God With us.
Go with the Comforter the Spirit of power and fire.
Go forth to liberate creation from oppression.
Go forth to heal and comfort God's people. Amen

Objects Symbols/objects/ideas: Certificate/token of recognition/appreciation, pebbles or any other appropriate or available symbols.

By Musa W. Dube

Part 5
Services on Social Factors Contributing to HIV/AIDS

1. Poverty and Economic Justice
   Leviticus 25:8-46 (Moiseraele P. Dibeele)
   Luke 16:19-31 (Tinyiko S. Maluleke)

2. Gender Injustice
   John 20:11-18 (Cheryl Dibeela)
   Joao 20:11-18 (Felicidade Cherinda)

3. Violence
   John 8:1-12 (Musa W. Dube)
   Judges 19 (Isabel Apawo Phiri)
   II Samuel 13:1-22 (Fulata L. Moyo)

4. Race and Ethnic Based Discrimination
   Genesis 21:8-21 (Augustine C. Musopule)
   Matthew 15:21-28 (Cheryl Dibeela)

5. Age Based Discrimination
   Mark 10:13-16 (Ezra Chitando)
   Genesis 18:1-15 (Isabel Apawo Phiri)

6. National Injustice
   Luke 4:16-22 (Ezra Chitando)

7. International Injustice
   Exodus 3:1-12 (Moiseraele P. Dibeele)

1. Poverty and Economic Justice

POVERTY AND ECONOMIC JUSTICE
Sermon Text: Leviticus 25:8-46

Introduction

This particular text is part of a large narrative called the holiness code, which covers Chapters 17 – 26 of the book of Leviticus. It is generally agreed that this discourse is a literary unit on its own, and has been incorporated into the book of Leviticus. The originators of this code were the priestly movement who were interested in ritual purity and temple worship. It is clear that they did not invent the code, but the document as it stands is a codification of customary law.

We Listen to the Word of God

DETAILS OF THE TEXT
Our text offers a radical economic system to the house of Israel. It prescribes a year of Jubilee in which a) the land shall lie fallow, b) the grains shall go un-harvested, c) the people shall return to their ancestral homes, d) there shall be fair trade, e) there shall be fidelity to the Torah/Law of Moses, f) people shall not make profit from the poor, g) and aliens shall be given hospitality. These covenantal prescriptions were meant to protect the poor and to safeguard the integrity of creation. It is an economic policy that has a bias towards the poor, orphans, widows, strangers and the weak. Such policies should inform us in our struggle against HIV/AIDS, which thrives through poverty, gender injustice, and the abuse of orphans and widows.

We Apply the Word of God to Ourselves and the Congregation

Many people build a wall between economics and theology, or shall we say faith reflection. They do not see the two relating, for the former is perceived to be about the mundane things of this of life, whilst the latter are about the heavenly things of God. As we see, this is refuted by our text.

WHAT CAN WE LEARN?
Africa has been riddled with poverty for many generations. The poverty breeds other related problems such as AIDS, corruption, greed and wars. However, our text envisages a situation of holistic social justice, where there is respect for God, for Creation, and for human beings. Yahweh requires just systems based on God's law, which is full of grace and mercy.

WHAT CAN WE CONFESS?
 We confess that:
- We tolerate structural injustice in our countries, which condemns millions of God's people to poverty;
- The church is often guilty of economic injustice by failing to pay just wages to its workers;
- We often fail to read God' s 'economic ordinances' contained in the Bible;
- We have not taken a prophetic role against our corrupt national governments.

WHAT CAN WE BE THANKFUL FOR?
We thank God for:
- God's word that is full of hope and provides signposts on how to live;
- The continent of Africa, its riches in raw materials, and its people;
- Those who run poverty eradication programs in our countries.

WHAT CAN WE PRAY FOR?

All: Kum ba yah my Lord,
            Kum ba yah (3x)
            Oh Lord! Kum ba yah.

Leader 1:   Someone is Crying Lord,
            Kum ba yah,

            Among the millions and in many places, there are tears of
            suffering, there are tears of weakness and disappointment. There are tears of
            strength and resilience. There are tears of the rich and tears of the poor.
            Someone is crying Lord, redeem the times.

All: Someone is dying Lord,
            Kum ba yah (3x)

Leader 2:   Some are dying of hunger and thirst; some are dying because others
            are enjoying unnecessary and superfluous things. Someone is dying
            because people go on exploiting one another. Some are dying because there are
            structures and systems which crush the poor and alienate the rich. Someone is
            dying Lord, because we are still not prepared to take a side, to make a choice, to
            be a witness. Someone is dying, Lord, redeem these times.

All: Someone is shouting Lord,
            Kum ba yah (3x)

Leader 3:   Someone is shouting out loud and clear. Someone has made a choice.
            Someone is ready to stand against the times. Someone is shouting out,
            offering their existence in love and anger to fight death surrounding us,
            to wrestle with the evil with which we crucify each other. Someone is shouting,
            Lord, redeem the times.

All: Someone is praying Lord,
            Kum ba yah (3x)

Leader 4:   Someone is praying Lord, we are praying in tears and anger
            in frustration and weakness, in strength and endurance,
            we are shouting and wrestling, as Jacob wrestled with the angel,
            and was touched, and was marked, and became a blessing,
            we are praying, Lord, spur our imagination, through Jesus Christ,

You have let us know where you want us to be.
Help us to be there now, be with us now, touch us, mark us,
Let us be a blessing. Let your power be present is our weakness,
Someone is praying Lord, redeem the times.

All: Kum ba yah my Lord,
Kum ba yah (3x)
Oh Lord kum ba yah. Amen
(© Negro Spiritual; *Prayers taken from God's future Today,*
London: CWM, 1987)

Suggested idea: The above is both a prayer and a song. It would be helpful to choose people ahead of time who would be the leaders. As they read out the words provided, the rest of the congregation would quietly hum the Kum ba yah tune. The prayers must be read out with conviction. Additional prayers could be written to go with these already provided.

By Moiseraele P. Dibeela

POVERTY AND DESTITUTION
Sermon Text: Luke 16: 19-31

Call to Worship
We recite the Song of Mary - Luke 1:46-55

My soul glorifies the Lord,
And my spirit rejoices in God my Savior,
For he has been mindful
Of the humble state of his servant.
From now on all generations will call me blessed,
For the Mighty One has done great things for me--
Holy is his name.
His mercy extends to those who fear him,
From generation to generation.
He has performed mighty deeds with his arm;
He has scattered those who are proud in their inmost thoughts.
He has brought down rulers from their thrones
But has lifted up the humble.
He has filled the hungry with good things
But has sent the rich away empty.
He has helped his servant Israel,
Remembering to be merciful
To Abraham and his descendants forever,
Even as he said to our fathers.
Amen

Song

An appropriate song about poverty or destitution may be sung, care must be taken to avoid songs that spiritualize poverty.

Introduction

Human beings have never been wealthier than they have become in our times. Ironically as wealth has grown in the world, so has inequality. Effectively therefore, we have on the one hand the growing wealth of the few, and the equally growing gap between the rich and the poor. It is estimated that up to one billion people in the world are unable to secure food and water. Needless to say, the majority of the world's poor are to be found in the two-thirds world. While HIV/AIDS is no respecter of persons, nations or races; it is true that people living in abject poverty are more susceptible to contacting the virus. Destitution and desperation leads many poor people to engage in risky sexual behavior, hence the HIV infection rate among the poor is higher. To state the matter in this way is not to offer an excuse for the poor and destitute, but to acknowledge an important reality. Apart from its role in the spread of HIV, poverty is in its own right, an abominable assault on human dignity. Poverty should therefore be combated as well. However we would be committing a serious omission if we did not point out the link between poverty and the spread of HIV/AIDS.

We Listen to the Word of God

We read Luke 16:19-31
DETAILS OF THE TEXT
This is one of the few judgment day parables. In this group of parables, Jesus portrays judgment day scenarios as a means of encouraging conversion in his listeners. Through these parables Jesus is able to demonstrate in concrete terms the kinds of behaviors, activities and attitudes necessary for finding favor on judgment day. It is a much more effective teaching tool than the simple listing of virtues and vices. Perhaps there is something of a lesson for HIV/AIDS prevention campaigners here. It may not be enough to proclaim long lists of virtuous and moral behaviors. It may be more effective to present credible and gripping scenarios.

In this parable we are told of the lives of two contemporaries, Lazarus and the rich man. Note the amazing literary feat of the storyteller. He names the poor man - Lazarus - and leaves the rich man unnamed. Elsewhere in the New Testament, it is often the prominent, rich males who are named, while the poor and female are not. Though Lazarus and the rich man were contemporaries living in the same city and village, and literally sharing the same living space - Lazarus lived at the rich man's gate, so that he smelt the food from the his kitchen and longed to eat what fell from the rich man's table - their lives could not have been more dissimilar. It seems that in that society, rich and poor lived side by side.

There was grinding poverty in the face of 'stinking' wealth. While the rich man was dressed in purple and fine linen, Lazarus' body was 'dressed' in open sores - so that the dogs came to lick the sores. Without clothes and malnourished, Lazarus was a perfect candidate for disease and premature death. While the rich man lived in luxury, Lazarus lived in abject poverty. How is it possible that their lives can be so markedly different? We cannot expect Lazarus to have matched the rich man's wealth pound for pound, but their contrasting fortunes are striking. The fact that it

223

was possible for the rich man to live in excess wealth, means that it was unnecessary for Lazarus to live in abject poverty. There was something wrong with the economic model that governed the city where they lived.

The story comes to a head when Lazarus and the rich man die and proceed to life after death. The rich man went straight to hell where he experiences torment, while the poor man is taken by angels to heaven where he sits by Abraham's side. The story gives the impression that Lazarus was admitted into heaven purely on the basis of his poverty, and the rich man was sent to hell purely on the basis of his wealth - suggestions that have caused a great deal of debate and controversy. It seems that the rich man had not only ignored the injunctions of Moses and the prophets during his lifetime, but had also failed to respond to the plight of Lazarus even as Lazarus stood at his gate. Herein lay the error of the rich man. As for poor Lazarus, he endured the indignity of his poverty with courage and tenacity, making his presence felt at the rich man's gates. In the sight of such opulence and such abundance he did not rise to plunder and rob, in the face of hunger and disease he did not force his way into the rich man's palace, in the face of being ignored daily he sat in hope at the gates of the rich man's home. This appears to be the reason he was rewarded.

We Apply the Word of God to Ourselves

WHAT CAN WE LEARN?
- That when massive poverty exists alongside massive wealth, there is something wrong with the socio-economic arrangements;
- That the inequality cannot be sustained without dire consequences in the long-term;
- That there is a definite linkage between susceptibility to HIV infection and poverty;
- Parabolic scenario based teaching may be more effective in HIV/AIDS prevention campaigns than moralizing.

WHAT DO WE HAVE TO CONFESS?
- We confess that we have not done enough to challenge policies that allow a few very wealthy people to live alongside many very poor people;
- We confess that in failing to eradicate poverty, we have contributed to the spread of HIV/AIDS;
- We confess that we moralize about HIV/AIDS instead of offering realistic real-life HIV/AIDS scenarios in our teaching about HIV/AIDS prevention.

WHAT CAN WE BE THANKFUL FOR?
- We can be thankful for the fact that the are poor people who have not succumbed to the indignities and temptations that come with poverty.
- We can be thankful that there are rich people who see the Lazaruses at their gates and are willing to look for long-term solutions.

WHAT CAN WE PRAY FOR?
- We pray for policy makers and economic planners to work for a world where there is a more equal distribution of wealth.

We Apply the Word of God to the Congregation

WHAT CAN WE FEEL?
- We should feel lucky that in a world where extremely rich and extremely poor live side by side with an ever widening gap, there has not been more conflict, more crime and more instability.

WHAT CAN WE BE?
- We can be activists in the eradication of poverty.

Conclusion: A Word to Society

How many other poor people will be able to endure the indignity of poverty, to smell delicious food from next door and not rise to demand, rob or plunder? How many poor people will not succumb to the temptation of selling their bodies and souls in exchange for a little food on the table? This is what makes poor people so susceptible to HIV/AIDS in our times. In this sense Lazarus is an exception who cannot be used as a role model. For many poor people are not able to wait for heavenly rewards. Yet even as the poor rise in protest and are forced to use survival tactics, they can only put themselves in further risk and danger.

Prayer of Commitment
Someone may recite Psalm 10:12-20

Arise, LORD! Lift up your hand, O God.
Do not forget the helpless.
Why does the wicked man revile God?
Why does he say to himself?
"He won't call me to account"?
But you, O God, do see trouble and grief;
You consider it to take it in hand.
The victim commits himself to you;
You are the helper of the fatherless.
Break the arm of the wicked and evil man;
Call him to account for his wickedness
That would not be found out.
The LORD is King for ever and ever;
The nations will perish from his land.
You hear, O LORD, the desire of the afflicted;
You encourage them, and you listen to their cry,
Defending the fatherless and the oppressed,
In order that man, who is of the earth, may terrify no more. Amen

Song
Choose any appropriate song

Symbols/objects: Food, sack clothes, fruits, gold, globe, broken wall, etc.

By Tinyiko S. Maluleke

2. Gender Injustice

GENDER INJUSTICE
Sermon Text: John 20:11-18

Introduction

Amongst all the developments achieved in Botswana society since independence -- namely development of economics and infrastructure – the one slow development is that of gender justice. This is not unique to Botswana, as gender injustice is common all over the world. In Botswana, however, some advancement has been made to address the inequalities experienced by women. Women's groups have mainly spearheaded these efforts.

In spite of the on going attempts, there are still a lot of inequalities experienced by women. Even though women make up 51% of the population of Botswana, their full legal capacity is being denied under both Common and Customary law in Botswana. Evidence suggests that certain provisions discriminate against women under these laws. This has led women to have fewer advantages culturally, socially, economically and sexually than their male counterparts. Men are believed to make decisions and determine the livelihood of everybody. This is true in all spheres of Botswana society: politics, the workplace, the home, and institutions like the Church. This has a direct impact and implication on the spread of HIV/AIDS and the role of caregivers, etc. Women have no control over their bodies. They can hardly say no to unprotected sex from their partners or husbands, even when they know that their partners are unfaithful. Women are also exposed to violence and rape. This makes them vulnerable to HIV/AIDS infection.

We Listen to the Word of God

DETAILS OF THE TEXT
I see the resurrection of Jesus as a symbol of freedom. Jesus' followers were relieved when they discovered that the body of Jesus was not there. Their sadness turned to joy, as they knew that death was not the ultimate for Jesus. Jesus' freedom inspired the disciples to feel the very freedom that he experienced; freedom from condemnation, and freedom from the pain of the crucifixion -- ultimate freedom. Jesus' freedom meant freedom for his followers. They had no reason to be frightened, hurt or depressed because Jesus was alive. He came to free all.

It is ironic that Mary being a woman is the bearer of this message of freedom, and experienced that ultimate freedom first. In fact, the other gospels mention Mary as being amongst other women. They were the ones that passed on this message of freedom to the rest of the male followers. This is ironic because women are the very ones bound by law, traditions and culture. They are the ones bound in relationships of violence and hurt and are the ones that are often too scared to spread this message of freedom to the rest of the society. Research indicates that gender injustice is one of the main contributors towards the spread of HIV/AIDS, and that if education is provided in this regard, the issue of gender inequality needs to be addressed as well. I believe this passage has a very important message for women as liberators of their own oppression.

We Apply the Word of God to Ourselves

WHAT CAN WE LEARN?
- That women ought to be the bearers of the message of freedom and gender justice and take responsibility not to get infected with HIV/AIDS;
- That women need to spearhead activities to liberate women;
- That Jesus Christ revealed himself to women and commissions them to tell the good news of his resurrection.

WHAT DO WE HAVE TO CONFESS?
- That we as women often fail to speak out and just accept the status quo;
- That women are sometimes guilty of oppressing themselves and other women further with their attitudes, infidelity and dishonesty;
- That as men, in families, church and society we have denied women the freedom God gives to them.

WHAT CAN WE BE THANKFUL FOR?
- For the many advancements made towards gender justice;
- That we worship a God of justice;
- For Jesus who went beyond traditions and cultures to achieve gender justice.

WHAT CAN WE PRAY FOR?
- For the elimination of the spread of HIV/AIDS that is fuelled by gender injustice;
- For women and men to become aware of gender injustice;
- For the Church which is guilty of perpetuating gender injustice;
- For the human rights as women's rights.

We Apply the Word of God to our Church/Society

WHAT CAN WE DO?
- We need deliberate educational strategies to educate people about gender injustice from a biblical perspective;
- To be prophetic and address issues around language, attitudes, culture and traditions when they come up in forums;
- Become strong advocates as men and women on gender justice.

Song
The leader may choose the appropriate song

Prayer
God our creator, your image is so beautiful. It may vary from child, to mother, from grandfather to lover, but it is your image.

We pray that we might see the same beautiful images in each other.
Help us to grow beyond our own prejudices of gender injustice, hatred and abuse.

Help us to appreciate our differences, so that we might affirm each other.
Mould us into your image, we pray. Amen

By Cheryl Dibeela

INJUSTICA BASEADA NO GENERO
Texto sugerido: João 20:11-18

Introdução

Entende-se por género o papel que a sociedade dá aos homens mulheres rapazes e raparigas. A injustiça do género refere-se ao facto de a sociedade não dar poder igual para homens e mulheres. Mulheres e raparigas são inferiorizadas, não são dadas os seus direitos, chegando ao cúmulo de na Bíblia não serem numericamente mencionadas (Mt 14.21). Essa discriminação faz com que elas sejam excluídas na execução de muitas tarefas, sobretudo nas de lidarença. Durante a sua vida terrena, Jesus notabilizou-se na defesa, integração e na restauração da dignidade da mulher. Na era do HIV/SIDA, as mulheres devem deixar de se esconder, de lamentar e de chorar, procurando informar-se cada vez mais e melhor sobre esta doença e estar na vanguarda no seu combate. Muitas vezes, as mulheres não têm poder para recusar o sexo, mesmo quando não estão preparadas. Isso faz delas escravas da vontade dos seus companheiros. Não à violência, não à violação, não à gravidez indesejada, não à infecção de qualquer género, não à discriminação. Em muitas culturas, as mulheres não tem poder para ser líderes mas, nesta passagem, Jesus dá à mulher poder para liderar. Se quisermos lutar contra o HIV/SIDA, as mulheres tem que ser dadas poder, como Jesus fez.

ORAÇÃO
Obrigada Senhor, por me teres feito mulher. Isso faz de mim, uma criatura doce, amável, delicada sem ser fraca, e aquela que traz novos seres ao mundo. Obrigada por me teres chamado ao teu serviço. Por causa dessa chamada, tenho muitas oportunidades de ajudar outras pessoas. Faça com que as mulheres tenham ouvidos para ouvir e olhos para ver, sobretudo no que diz respeito ao HIV/SIDA. Amen

CANÇÂO
Escolhe uma que esteja de acordo com a mensagem

Você sabia que quando,
A fotografia da família está na secretária DELE
Ah! Ele é um homem de família sólida e responsável.
A fotografia da família está na secretária DELA
Humm, a sua família é mais importante do que a sua carreira.

A mesa DELE está desordenada. Ele é um homem trabalhador e muito ocupado.
A mesa DELA está desordenada. Ela é obviamente muito desorganizada.

ELE está a falar com os colegas. De certeza está a discutir assuntos do serviço.
ELA está a falar com as colegas. Deve estar a fazer fofoca!

228

ELE não está na sua secretária, deve estar numa reunião.
ELA não está na sua secretária. Deve estar na casa de banho.

ELE está a almoçar com o director da empresa, de certeza que vai ser promovido
ELA está a almoçar com o director da empresa, devem ter um caso.

ELE vai a uma conferência internacional. É bom para a sua carreira.
ELA vai a uma conferência internacional. O que é que o marido vai dizer?

ELE vai fazer o seu doutoramento. È bom para a sua carreira.
ELA vai fazer o seu doutoramento. O que é que ela quer provar?

ELE vai sair para um trabalho melhor. Ele sabe reconhecer uma boa oportunidade.
ELA vai sair para um trabalho melhor. Não se pode depender das mulheres.

Autor anônimo (a)

Por: Felicidade N. Cherinda

3. Violence

VIOLENCE AGAINST WOMEN
Suggested Passage: John 8:1-12

Instructions: By using the poetic opening, lead the congregation to grasp the reality of violence against women through the various stories of biblical women and the women in our lives, many of whom undergo violence. Assign different verses to different women and let them read their verses wherever they are seated. The poetic opening will be followed by the reading of the text. Given that violence is often shrouded in silence, arrange in advance for one woman to stand up and retell the story of the woman caught in adultery, explaining or providing missing information. If time and setting does not allow, begin with the introduction going downward or use some of the poetic verses. The leader may use some of the suggested symbols to arrange the meeting place accordingly.

Poetic Opening

Woman 1:	I am Eve, the bone of your bone, and the flesh of your flesh.
Woman 2:	I am Sarah, the woman who calls you Lord and master.
Woman 3:	I am Hagar your maidservant; your unofficial wife.
Woman 4:	I am Leah, the woman you married against your will.
Woman 5:	I am Dinah your only daughter who is raped by Schechem.
Woman 6:	I am Tamar, your desperate widow who plays the sex worker.
Woman 7:	I am Ruth, your widow sleeping at your feet, asking for your cover.
Woman 8:	I am Bathsheba, raped and married by your king.
Woman 9:	I am Vashti, your wife killed so that all women may obey husbands.
Woman 10:	I am the Levite's concubine, raped by the mob and cut up by my lover.

229

All Women:	We are the broken women of the Hebrew Bible.
	We are the broken women in a broken world.
	We are women searching for our own healing.
Woman 11:	I am Mary, the pregnant woman with no place to go.
Woman 12:	I am the Samaritan woman, with five husbands and none for her own.
Woman 13:	I am Martha, the woman who is cooking while you sit and talk.
Woman 14:	I am Mary, the woman who silently anoints your feet with oil.
Woman 15:	I am the street woman, washing your feet with my tears.
Woman 16:	I am the bent over woman, waiting for your healing touch.
Woman 17:	I am the bleeding woman, struggling to touch your garment of power.
Woman 18:	I am Anna, the widow praying for liberation in your church.
Woman 19:	I am the persistent widow in your courts, crying, "Grant me Justice."
Woman 20:	I am Jezebel, the demonized woman, blamed for all evil.
All Women:	We are women of the New Testament.
	We are broken women in a broken world.
	We are women searching for our own healing.
Woman 21:	I am the woman in your home, I am your wife.
Woman 22:	I am the woman in your house, I am your lover, your live-in girlfriend.
Woman 23:	I am the woman in your life, I am your mother.
Woman 24:	I am a woman in your workplace, I am your secretary.
Woman 25:	I am a woman in your streets, I am your sex worker.
Woman 26:	I am a working woman in your house with no property of my own.
Woman 27:	I am the woman in your life with no control over my body.
Woman 28:	I am the woman in your bed with a blue eye and broken ribs.
Woman 29:	I am the woman raped in your house, streets, offices and church.
Woman 30:	I am the woman in your church, cooking, cleaning, clapping and dancing.
All Women:	We are women of the world.
	We are African Women.
	And we are Christian women.
	We are broken women in a broken world.
	We are women seeking for our own healing.

Introduction

Violence against women takes many different forms and can be emotional, physical, psychological and economic. In most cases, it is closely linked with gender inequalities, which deny women control over their bodies, leadership and economic power. In the HIV/AIDS era, violence against women hampers both HIV/AIDS prevention and provision of quality care to the infected. Sexual activities that are violent increase infection rates since the chance of bodily tearing is high. Further, in violent relationships women are often not able to insist on safer sex, or even abstinence. Further, the context of HIV/AIDS in itself has increased violence against women, since the girl child is targeted for rape by older men who believe they are less likely to be infected, and by HIV positive men who want to cleanse themselves of the virus. Women in stable relationships often find themselves blamed for bringing HIV/AIDS home and for witchcraft after the death of their spouses. They are dispossessed at the death of their spouses, forcing some to turn to sex work.

In many cultures, violence against women is tolerated in different ways. Some cultures think it is acceptable that husbands physically discipline their wives or partners. Some cultural perspectives lead friends and relatives to counsel abused women to endure and tolerate the violence. Church ministers ask abused women to forgive and submit to their abusing partners. Some countries have laws that make women second citizens and minors. All these are the structures that maintain and perpetuate violence against women.

Reading of the Text: John 8:1-12

Breaking the silence: Retell what happened to the accused woman; why the involved man was not brought forward, use contextual experiences and stories.

We Listen to the Word of God

DETAILS OF THE TEXT
Verses 1-2:
  - ➤ The setting of the story is given, both of place (Mount of Olives and temple courts) and the time (dawn). The setting gives us the background of where the story occurs.
  - ➤ The verses also highlight that there were many people around Jesus, who are witnesses to the woman's case. They also indicate that Jesus was a teacher.

Verses 3-4:
  - ➤ The woman caught in adultery, her accusers, the teachers of the law, and the Pharisees arrive in the temple. They state the case. She was caught in adultery and by the Law of Moses, she should be stoned. Note that they did not bring the man who was involved with her!
  - ➤ Note that she is made to stand before the whole group. Is this for embarrassment, or that she may be seen by all?
  - ➤ Note that her accusers, like Jesus, are teachers of the law and they base their case on the Law of Moses, either as written or as they interpret it. For some reason, they want Jesus' opinion, "Now what do you say?"
  - ➤ Note also that the woman does not speak for herself. She neither denies nor confirms. Her gender did not allow her to speak in court, as she was held to be a minor.

Verses 6-7:
  - ➤ The text gives us the reason for their question—they wanted to accuse Jesus, if he contradicts the law. Is this right to use a woman for their own arguments? This brings other questions to the fore: was she really caught in adultery, or set up and raped?
  - ➤ Note that Jesus, sensing their motive, keeps quite. Instead of making any verbal response, he starts to write on the ground with his finger. Why this silence? Is he thinking? Does he want them to think more about their case?

231

➤ Note that they persist, 'They kept on questioning him.' Then he responds. His response is not so much on quoting the Law of Moses, but on the basis of sin.

➤ Highlight that Jesus says they can stone her if they do not have any sin. It is not clear which sin Jesus refers too, but this may very well include adultery on the side of her accusers. It may not, but the point is every sin is sin, and no one is sinless.

➤ Highlight that Jesus challenges these leaders to realize that sin is sin regardless of who commits it. It should not be gendered. Jesus challenges them to apply law to both genders. Underline that women's sins are no worse that men's sins. Such a division sanctions the oppression of women.

Verses: 8-9:
➤ Jesus bends down again to write on the ground, giving his listeners time to reflect on what he said and time to examine themselves.

➤ Highlight the impact; namely, that the accusers leave, one by one. They realize they are also sinners. Such a point is important in the HIV/AIDS era where many church leaders have labeled those who are HIV positive are sinners who deserve punishment. Underline that those who are sinless be the first to label HIV positive people as deserving punishment. We are all sinful, only saved by grace.

➤ Highlight, "beginning with the elders," which indicates that many outstanding church leaders are not sinless. No one is sinless.

Verse 10-11:
➤ Jesus speaks to the woman and she speaks to him. Note that Jesus allows the woman to speak and assures her, "Neither do I condemn you.' This is grace. The latter is an important approach, for too many church leaders and relatives who receive abused women, condemn them. They stand with the accusers, by insisting that women must be obedient and humble, or that the victim invited it upon themselves.

➤ Highlight that Jesus refuses to side with the woman's accusers, who use her as a public spectacle, and are using the woman to trap him.

➤ Underline that Jesus, though himself sinless, does not condemn the woman. This point needs emphasis, for too many Christians who suppose themselves holy, rush to judge and to condemn those whom they regard as sinful. Our call as Christ's followers is to give grace. Like Jesus, we must not condemn anyone.

We Apply the Word of God to Ourselves

WHAT CAN WE LEARN?
• It is easy to be religious people who participate in violence against women;
• That in many societies women may not even have a chance to speak for themselves;
• That the interpretation of the law by male teachers can be biased against women;
• Many cultures, including the Bible, disregard men's sins and highlight those of women. This does not help us in the HIV/AIDS struggle;
• We can stand and advocate for the rights of the oppressed, including abused women.

WHAT DO WE HAVE TO CONFESS?
• We have not always stood against violence against women;
• Violence against women happens in our churches;

- Many Christian homes are violent against women;
- Many pastors' counseling of couples actually tolerates violence and is gender biased;
- Our tolerance for violence has not helped HIV/AIDS prevention and care.

WHAT CAN WE BE THANFUL FOR?
- The example that Jesus sets for us to resist violence against women;
- The biblical belief that all people were created in God's image;
- For grace that enables us to love, forgive and avoid being judgmental;
- The NGOs that fight violence against women;
- The human rights charters and the CEDAW convention.

WHAT CAN WE PRAY FOR?
- To become non-violent homes, Christian families and churches;
- To become a non-violent nation that protects the rights of women.

We Apply the Word of God to the Congregation

- We can promote the Decade of Overcoming Violence;
- Train our members on conflict resolution skills;

Conclusion: A Word on the Society

In many societies and homes, women are subjugated to violence on the basis of their gender. Unfortunately, many church structures and homes are not exemplary since they practice the culture of gender inequalities. Yet the gospel of Christ continues to challenge us to renew ourselves and to seek ever more to understand Christ and God's will for the world and all people. On this basis, we do well as a church to proclaim for ourselves and for the society at large that, "In Christ, there is neither male nor female" (Galatians 3:28), we are made in God's image (Genesis 1:27-28).

Song
Let us break bread together

Lord's Supper
Should be served as part of the healing.

Song
Ndi Mitima
(Thuma Mina, No. 14)
Or any other appropriate song.

Closing Prayer
Creator God, you created the earth and everything in it.
You created everything interdependent and you created everything good.
You created women and men in your image, you blessed them both.
Help us to see your image on the faces of the victims of our violence.

Help us to remember we have no right to subject anyone to violence.
Help all of us who live in violence to realize and to affirm our own dignity
Help us to realize we were made in God's image.
Help us to remember that we should never tolerate violence.
Help your church to realize that Jesus did not tolerate violence against women.
Help us to fight violence in the HIV/AIDS era, for it hampers both prevention and the provision of quality care. In Jesus name, we pray. Amen

Suggested Objects/symbols/ideas: Pictures of women in various situations; a testimony or a story of a woman who lived in violence and overcame it. Bread and wine for the Eucharist. You can invite someone who works with an NGO that deals with violence against women to give a brief talk on the issue.
By Musa W. Dube

VIOLENCE: RAPED ANDCUT INTO PIECES
Sermon Text: Judges 19

Prayer
By all

When God created the world, it was good. We gather together to affirm the goodness of the world that God created. We reclaim the good that is in all humanity. We reject the negative forces that bring pain and death in the life of the community. We claim the Spirit of God that brings renewal on earth so that justice can prevail. Amen

Song (Chichewa)
Singa anadula Yesu // (Chains were broken by Jesus)
Singa anadula, Yesu // (Chains were broken by Jesus)
Singa anadula // (Chains were broken)
Singa anadula // (Chains were broken)

Moyo wapereka, Yesu // (Life has been given by Jesus)
Moyo wapereka, Yesu // (Life has been given by Jesus)
Moyo wapereka // (Life has been given)
Moyo wapereka//(Life has been given)

Tiimbe Haleluya, Yesu // (We sing Haleluya, Jesus)
Tiimbe Haleluya, Jesu // (We sing Haleluya, Jesus)
Tiimbe Haleluya // (We sing Haleluya)
Tiimbe Haleluya // (We sing Haleluya) (A Popular Malawian Chorus)

Introduction

Domestic violence is one form of the gender-based violence experienced by women and girls in their homes. It occurs in the form of battery, sexual abuse of female children and workers, female genital mutilation, dowry-related violence, marital rape, emotional, verbal, psychological, economic and spiritual abuse. Domestic violence can lead to the hospitalization or even death of the victim. In the era of HIV/AIDS, domestic violence also leads to intentional infection of the victim with HIV.

Whatever form it takes, domestic violence makes women and girls live in the context of fear every day of their lives. The victims suffer physically, emotionally, psychologically and spiritually for a long time, especially where there are no support systems. When women and girls live in such a state, it has negative effect on the development of the society as a whole. Domestic violence is a common event suffered by a large number of women regardless of race, educational background and economic status. Women under such conditions cannot insist on safer sex, in or outside of wedlock. Neither can such women abstain or insist on faithfulness from their partners.

We Listen to the Word of God

The leader or a member of the congregation can read the text of Judges 19.
The story of Judges 19 is very shocking in its contents because of the way the concubine was treated, first by the owner of the house, and second by the Levite.

DETAILS OF THE TEXT
- ➢ There was a domestic problem that made the concubine of the Levite return to her father's house in Bethlehem. In the traditional African concept of marriage, the concubine would have been called one of the many wives of the Levite.
- ➢ The Levite followed his wife to her father's house to seek reconciliation.
- ➢ The father of the wife is happy about the prospect of reconciliation because in the Jewish culture, just like in the African culture, it is a disgrace for a woman to return to her parents due to marital problems. The father keeps the Levite much longer than he had intended. He seems hesitant about letting his daughter go.
- ➢ When the Levite started to return to his home in Judah with his wife, it was late and he had to seek night accommodation for himself, his wife and their party at an old man's home in Gibeah in Benjamin.
- ➢ In the evening, the men of Gebeah surrounded the old man's house demanding that they be able to rape the Levite his men.
- ➢ The old man found the request to be disgraceful. Instead he offered to let the men rape the wife of the Levite.
- ➢ The woman was thrown to the men outside and they raped her until morning. In the morning she was found dead outside the old man's house.
- ➢ The Levite took the body of his wife to Judah and on reaching home, he cut his wife's body into twelve peaces, which he sent to the twelve tribes of Israel, seeking revenge for the death of his wife.

We Apply the Word of God to Ourselves

WHAT CAN WE LEARN?

- Married women are under pressure to return to their husbands because they are not welcomed in their parents' home;
- Marriages where there are more than one wife have the potential of bringing HIV infection to the whole family, and in our period in the history of humanity they should be condemned;
- It is inhuman to give a woman to a mob of men to be raped, especially because one is protecting a man from rape;
- It is even more injustice to seek revenge for the murder of this woman, when one did not protest before she was given to the mob to be raped;
- Even if the woman would have survived the mob rape, if it was today, she could have been infected with HIV and she could have had serious psychological and emotional problems in her marriage and life.

WHAT CAN WE CONFESS?

- Not protecting married women from domestic violence;
- Choosing to protect men at the expense of women, especially in our counseling of couples who are having marital problems;
- Valuing the institution of marriage more than protecting the lives of abused married women;
- Turning a blind eye to the infidelity of married men in the name of culture, and yet being ruthless with the infidelity of married women;
- Keeping quiet when the institutionalized rape of married women is taking place through cleansing rituals;
- Tolerating patriarchal cultures that do not value women lives.

WHAT CAN WE BE THANKFUL FOR?

- That God is on the side of the suffering women;
- That God demands justice for all the oppressed people;
- There are church related organizations that provide shelter for abused women.

WHAT CAN WE PRAY FOR?

- All women who are in situations of abuse by their spouses;
- All the perpetrators of domestic violence to stop and start respecting women as human beings who reflect the image of God;
- The church to preach against domestic violence and to counsel couples in such a way that promotes justice;
- More church based institutions that work for the protection of abused married women;
- Church leaders to use their position to speak against domestic violence with their congregation and society at large.

We Apply the Word of God to the Congregation

WHAT CAN WE FEEL?
- Repentant that rape cases of wives are found even in Christian homes, and are justified by the wrong use of scriptures.
- Sorry for the married women whose future is ruined because of institutionalized rape after the death of her husband, when they are forced into cultural cleansing sexual rituals.
- Responsible for keeping quiet when rape was happening even with our knowledge.
- Anger towards the rapists, who are empowered by cultural beliefs and practices.

WHAT CAN WE BE?
- A community that is against any form of abuse against women and children;
- A healing community for victims and perpetrators of domestic violence.

WHAT CAN WE DO?
- Preach against violence towards children and women. We need to break the chains of silence;
- Provide shelter and counseling for victims of rape. Let us begin by creating an atmosphere of trust so that the victims can have the courage to talk about it;
- We also need to declare a zero tolerance for any form of abuse;
- We need to be open enough to accommodate the perpetrators of abuse. Confronting them alone will not solve the problem, we need to lead them to deliverance. We know Jesus as the one who delivers us from all forms of evil;
- We need to give back to people a sense of integrity and a purpose for life that is taken away by abuse;
- Train our church leaders on how to deal with domestic violence.

Conclusion: A Word on Society

The process of eradicating domestic violence requires a united approach. Individually, Christians need to make a commitment to stop domestic violence, starting with themselves and the members of their families. The community has the responsibility of stopping the cultural beliefs and practices that promote violence against women. At a church level, sermons that promote violence against women must stop. The church should not promote marriage at the expense of the lives of women. The community and the church need to accept the fact that sometimes divorce is necessary to preserve the lives of women from physical violence that could lead to death and exposure to the HIV. At a family level, there should be room and support for married women who return home because they are suffering from violence. At a national level, the constitution should have strict laws against the abuse of women, and the courts should be women friendly in their passing of sentences to perpetrators of domestic violence. Where such instruments are lacking, the church should assume a prophetic role to the society.

Prayer

By all

We the church of Jesus Christ confess that we have contributed to domestic violence by keeping quiet when we saw it happening, and by promoting teachings and practices that put the lives of married women in danger.

We seek your forgiveness Lord. We pray for courage to promote justice for both men and women. We thank you because if we confess our sins and we are sincere about it, you are willing to forgive us and help us to start a new life of justice and peace.
In Jesus name. Amen

Sharing the Peace

The congregation will share peace either by signing or saying the following words:

> Peace to you.
> We bless you now
> In the name of the Lord,
> Peace to you.
> We bless you now in the name of the prince,
> Peace to you.

Object/symbols/ideas: The preacher can organize a drama or concert that castigates all the acts of domestic violence, a broken reed or branch, a broken jaw bone, a sign of danger, a red light, blood soaked clothes, fallen teeth, broken ribs, musical instruments, etc.

By Isabel Apawo Phiri

TAMAR RAPED AT HOME
Sermon Text: II Samuel 13:1-22

Introduction

Jewish communities were kinship-based. It is a known reality that in such kinship-based communities, women learn from an early age to subordinate their own well being for the good of the community. In such communities, sexuality issues are power issues. Those who determine the 'what, when, where and how' of heterosexual sex are those who have power— in this case, men (Gupta 2001). Women cannot make sexual decisions and neither can they negotiate safer nor more honorable sex. Within such realities, even when virginity is demanded from girls, they have no power to determine this state. This was Tamar's reality.

Tragically the HIV/AIDS epidemic has fueled rape in Southern Africa. Rape cases have rocketed to epidemic levels in the past seven years as the HIV/AIDS epidemic grew. Why? There are many reasons. The epidemic's impact renders men powerless. They loose control—even over women's bodies. Now they are told to use condoms, to be faithful and to abstain! They are told to fear HIV/AIDS. Also women's bodies have always been associated with disease and seen to be the cause of men's disease. Not surprisingly, one on the reasons that rape has escalated is because it is believed that sleeping with a virgin cleanses one of HIV/AIDS! But what happens to the virgin? How does she cleanse herself? This is not a factor—she is after all a woman, and her body is there for men's service. She can die, I suppose. It does not matter. But some rape cases are also fueled by anger and revenge. Men who are HIV positive blame women for giving them sexually transmitted diseases (STDS). In fact many cultures in Southern Africa equate STDs with women. All these gendered perspectives only fuel violence against women and expose women to HIV/AIDS infection. Let us turn to the biblical text to view the case of Tamar's rape.

We Listen to the Word of God

Tamar was a beautiful girl, a virgin daughter of King David. Amnon was her stepbrother who had lustful feelings for his beautiful stepsister. Like most of our communities today, there were double standards when it came to sexual morality among the Jews. While virginity among girls was highly valued and expected, the expectations were different when it came to boys. Put the following questions to the audience:

- What cultural biases were Jonadab, Amnon's friend and cousin counting on when he gave the advice, which was to give a chance for Amnon to rape Tamar?
- Was Amnon fulfilled after raping Tamar? What feelings were experienced by Amnon, Tamar, David, Absalom (Tamar's brother)? Why?
- Why did David not punish Amnon after hearing that he had defiled Tamar?

DETAILS OF THE TEXT
In classic Greek, there were four words that could express the concept of love or affection. These were: **Eros**: meaning 'sexual attraction'; **Philia**: meaning 'brotherly/sisterly love'; **Storge**: meaning 'family affection' and **Agape**: meaning 'self-giving' love. What Amnon felt for Tamar in verse 1 of our Biblical texts cannot be defined as love in its true sense (an attitude of affection and goodwill that respects the loved- not uncontrolled emotions), but lust, so probably a very selfish *eros* by one person without any respect for the other?

Verses 1-2:
➤ Amnon thinks he is in love with his stepsister Tamar. He knows she is a virgin and therefore a girl with very high sexual morality, and so principled that she cannot be coaxed into have sexual intercourse with him.

Verses 3-8:
➤ Amnon takes his sexist friend's advice and acts on it. He deceives his father David and even Tamar. David who himself who had raped Bathsheba and deceived Uriah and the rest of his people, lived to see the same (plus incest) happen within his family –(in fulfillment of God's judgment through Nathan's pronouncements?)

Verse 12-14:
➤ Tamar was aware of the double standard of sexual expectations amongst their people. When Tamar tried to reason with him about the humiliating results of sex outside marriage, Amnon used force and raped her.

Verse 15-19:
➤ What seemed to be love clearly turned out to be lust? After raping her, Amnon hated her. She was so violated and humiliated that servants had to shut her out in obedience to their

master's directive. She had lost her virginity and therefore had to tear the richly ornamented robe she had been wearing.

Verses 20-22:
➢ Absalom took her in, offering consolation while concealing his own hatred for Amnon.

We Apply the Word of God to Ourselves

WHAT CAN WE LEARN?
• True love respects the wishes and desires of the person it targets but anything less than that is selfish and violating; lustful feelings that should not be entertained in any way.

WHAT CAN WE CONFESS?
• Abusing our powers so as to violate other people's freedoms and rights;
• Contributing to an environment that makes those we consider powerless, live with no control over their bodies;
• Condoning a culture of abuse of the powerless (especially women and children) by our silence and fear, thus making them more vulnerable to sexually transmitted infections including HIV.

WHAT CAN WE BE THANKFUL FOR?
• We have a model of what love should be in God's love for us, male and female;
• There are clear laws against violence towards women; especially rape.

WHAT CAN WE PRAY FOR?
• That both men and women will be committed to fight against violence against women.
• The Church will be prophetic, even in issues of gender disparity that lead to violence against women.
• That women in abusive sexual relationships will denounce these practices by coming out in the open against the abuser, and by refusing to continue in such relationships that make them less than what God intended for them.

WHAT CAN WE FEEL?
• Anger at the people who practice such abuses;
• Compassion for the women who have experienced such abuses;
• Concern for the rape victim's well being (psychological, as well as physical).

WHAT SHOULD WE BE?
• A healing community that is committed to making better living conditions for every member of the community- making sure that there is fair distribution of power.

WHAT CAN WE DO?
• Preaching and teaching sexuality education that emphasizes mutuality and respect;
• Denounce any form of violence, including rape;
• Report any known cases of violence against women and children.

We Apply the Word of God to the Congregation and Society

- The Church should refuse to wed any couples that have not been counseled about the mutuality and respect of each partner in a marriage relationship, especially in this HIV/AIDS era.
- We must denounce the double standard of sexual morality, in both the Church and community at large- acknowledging that sexual abstinence and faithfulness is expected from both men and woman.
- The Church should put pressure on governments to take tougher actions against rapists and provide counseling for victims.

WE PREACH THE GOSPEL
"Love is patient, love is kind. It does not envy, it does not boast, it is not proud. It is not rude, it is not self-seeking, it is not easily angered, and it keeps no record of wrongs. Love does not delight in evil but rejoices with truth. It always protects…" (I Corinthians 13:4-7).

Song
What a friend we have in Jesus

Closing Prayer
Your body was broken for us. Your blood was spilled for us. We as women have been washed clean and made members of your body through baptism. We are the temples of your Holy Spirit. Help us to remember this and to refuse to tolerate any violence against us. Help us to say no to HIV/AIDS death. Bless us Lord, Amen.

All: The grace of our Savoir Jesus Christ, the love of God and the fellowship of the Holy Spirit remain with us all, now and ever more. **AMEN**

By Fulata L. Moyo

4. Race and Ethnic Based Discrimination

RACE-BASED DISCRIMINATION
Sermon Text: Genesis 21:8-21

Introduction

The theme of discrimination is central to this story. Hagar is from Egypt, while Abraham and Sarah are from Ur of the Chaldeans. One is a servant and the other master/mistress, their power relations are not the same and it becomes part of the problem. They did not speak the same language and did not have the same culture. However, when Hagar gave birth to Ishmael as a surrogate for Sarah, it affected the power relations and made Sarah bitter. The two women were both victims of a patriarchal society. Nowadays discrimination is based on many things and it is not limited to gender. Discrimination against those who are HIV positive is very prevalent today. It takes place on personal, cultural, economic and community levels. The children also suffer as orphans who are often ill-treated or exploited by guardians.

God has to work with us, as our cultural conditioning more often than not, gets into God's way. What God promises, God fulfills in God's own time and way. In and through God's activity, God also reveals who God is. God never gives up on God's own people even those who have resulted from human mistakes. We need to learn to accept our mistakes and live with their consequences, even as God continues to bless us.

We Listen to the Word of God

The story of the relationship between Sarah and Hagar is a tragedy and all involved are victims. The God of impossibilities left it too long to tempt both Abraham and Sarah to try to fulfill the promise of a child. Very few of us could have behaved differently. Seeking to fulfill the cultural expectation of fatherhood and motherhood through a surrogate sexual partner was such a powerful force that Abraham and Sarah succumbed to the temptation with devastating consequences for all. What can we learn from this story about all involved, including God?

Consider the following questions:
- What caused Sarah to request Abraham to get rid of Hagar and her son?
- What did Sarah fear? Why was Abraham distressed?
- Who gets hurt by discrimination?
- Did God's intervention in both cases change the situation in any way?

We Apply the Word of God to Ourselves and the Congregation

WHAT CAN WE LEARN?
- That child bearing was, and still is, considered critical to being fulfilled as a woman or man in many cultures;
- That we are often influenced by cultural norms in our decisions and these may be contrary to the will of God;

- That mistakes may have long term consequences for all involved;
- That God may intervene in the consequences of our mistakes and continue to bless us. This is grace.

WHAT CAN WE CONFESS?
- Being self-centred and using other people;
- Causing pain to others and refusing to accept responsibility;
- Men's sexual sins in the name of culture;
- Putting pressure on women to bear heirs;
- That the expectation to parent makes HIV/AIDS prevention difficulties;
- Discriminating against women.

WHAT CAN WE BE THANKFUL FOR?
- God's unfailing promises;
- God's loving intervention and blessings;
- That all were created in God's image.

WHAT CAN WE PRAY FOR?
- Wisdom to decide well;
- God's forgiveness when we make mistakes;
- The capacity to live peacefully with our differences.

WHAT CAN WE FEEL?
- Sympathy for Hagar and Ishmael;
- Sorry for Sarah and Abraham for the cultural pressure they under went;
- Happiness at God's intervention.

WHAT CAN WE BE?
- Trustful of God's promises;
- Loving to other people in the community;
- Parents for the many orphaned children.

WHAT CAN WE DO?
- Identify those who are being discriminated against in our communities;
- Take action to address the problem communally, by creating awareness and providing physical and legal protection;
- Provide care for those who are suffering from HIV/AIDS, or suffering as a consequence of it;
- Adopt children orphaned by HIV/AIDS.

Put these questions to the congregation:
- Did Sarah do the right thing?
- Who gets hurt by the discrimination we practice it against others?
- What can we learn from God's intervention?
- Would you have done differently if you were Abraham?
- What are some of the cultural practices that people follow, but are contrary to God's word?

We Apply the Word of God to the Congregation

- What did Sarah and Hagar not have in common?
- What role did class and racial distinctions play in their difficult relationship?
- How do we deal positively with distinctions of class, gender, and race in the congregations?
- How can we celebrate difference among ourselves?

Song
What a Friend we have in Jesus

What a friend we have in Jesus,
All our sins and grieves to bear!
What a privilege to carry,
Everything to God in prayer!
O what peace we often forfeit!
O what needless pain we bear!
All because we do not carry
Everything to God in prayer.

Have we trials and temptations?
Is there trouble anywhere?
We should never be discouraged;
Take it to the Lord in prayer.
Can we find a friend so faithful,
Who will all our sorrows share?
Jesus knows our every weakness;
Take it to the Lord in prayer.

Are we weak and heavy-laden,
Cumbered with a load of care?
Precious Savior still our refuge,
Take it to the Lord in prayer.
Do they friends despise, forsake thee?
Take it to the Lord in prayer;
In His arms He'll take and shield thee,
Thou wilt find a solace there.

(© Joseph Medlicott Scriven (1820-86), Hymns of Faith No. 461)

Prayer
Read Psalm 103 responsively or any appropriate prayer.

Suggested Objects/symbols/ideas: Walking stick, suitcase, ticket, barrier, poster of refugees or displaced persons, chains, etc.   By Augustine C. Musopule

ETHNIC DISCRIMINATION
Sermon Text: Matthew 15:21-28

Introduction

Ethnic discrimination has always been part of Southern Africa and other parts of Africa. We grew up believing that other cultural groups were either better or worse than ourselves. This has not died down. Having lived in South Africa, Botswana and England, I have come across conversations in which derogatory terms are used for people from different ethnic backgrounds. In some countries this discrimination has increased to the extent that ethnic wars have developed between people. Does this apply to your own context, country and region?

Today with a lot of instability in countries surrounding Botswana, people from other ethnic groups are flooding the country hoping to find a better life. This has resulted in xenophobia on the part of the locals, and one can say that we adopt the same discriminatory attitude portrayed in the passage. These attitudes are not only prevalent against foreigners, but also exercised within the country against the ethnic minority groups themselves. The disadvantages are always conspicuous on the side of the groups discriminated against. With HIV/AIDS, for example, these are the groups that would have less educational opportunities; they are the ones that would not have easy access to Anti-retroviral drugs or medical care. They are often the ones left behind when any advancements are made. As for immigrants, they often have no legal right to health services, jobs and education and this does not help in both prevention and care.

We Listen to the Word of God

DETAILS OF THE TEXT

The prejudice, which the Jews felt toward the Syrophoenician woman, is clear in the passage. Matthew calls her Canaanite, an indication that she comes from a people of reproach. It is Jesus' attitude that surprises me and makes the story difficult to understand, since he is usually the one who does not harbor discriminatory attitudes. Jesus, in other stories, like with the Samaritan woman (John 4), crosses boundaries and reaches out to people in spite of the Jewish expectations and beliefs to stay away from other ethnic groups.

In this passage, however, he approaches the woman with harshness and prejudice. He first of all implies that he has not come for any people, except the Jews. He also uses the derogatory term which was used at the time for people who were believed to have been godless – namely dogs. He uses the diminutive term 'puppies' or 'doggies'. Some commentaries believe he was just being humoristic, whilst others say that he wanted to teach his followers a lesson. To me, it seems that Jesus' own prejudices were tested. The woman's faith and persistence opened Jesus' eyes. This is in itself is very good. If Jesus could change his views about discrimination, we should also do the same.

We Apply the Word of God to Ourselves

WHAT CAN WE LEARN?
- That Jesus' prejudices to other cultural groups were also tested and that we are not immune to such prejudices;
- Jesus was willing to change his mind.

WHAT DO WE HAVE TO CONFESS?
- That we are most of the time guilty of ethnic discrimination;
- That we have referred to some ethnic groups as dogs;
- That we have refused to talk to some ethnic groups;
- That we have served only our own people.

WHAT CAN WE BE THANKFUL FOR?
- That God created us with diverse languages, colors and cultures;
- That we are all created in God's image;
- That all the children deserve bread at the table.

WHAT CAN WE PRAY FOR?
- That we might open up and accept people who are different from us;
- That all people should get equal access to medical facilities and HIV/AIDS treatment despite who they are or where they come from;
- That international pharmacies will make HIV/AIDS drugs affordable for all people.

We Apply the Word of God to our Church/Society

WHAT CAN WE DO?
- Partner with groups that are different from us so as to learn about their cultures;
- Lobby for HIV/AIDS medical services on behalf of disadvantaged and discriminated groups and for immigrants;
- Provide education to groups so that they might learn about other cultures and have the opportunity to ask questions and understand;
- Fight the HIV/AIDS stigma and discrimination against people living with HIV/AIDS (PLWHA's).

Illustration
The text is rewritten to highlight some of the ways in which we discriminate today.

Verse 21:
- ➤ In order to avoid any further interruption at the surgery, the doctor decided to go home. He got into his car and drove off to find some quiet time.

Verse 22:
- ➤ However, as he approached his gate he found a refugee sitting and waiting. Tearfully the woman said: 'Please help me. My child is very sick and I have no money.'

Most refugees leave their countries to come and find a better life elsewhere,
Especially now that the economic situation has become unbearable with no
basic necessities and no medical facilities in their home countries.

Verse 23:
> He just ignored the woman and drove past her into the garage. Just then a neighbor came out and encouraged him to send her off. 'Send her away, she is just making a nuisance of herself. They are all the same'.

Verse 24:
> He said to the woman. 'There are many of our own people who have need of help'.

Verse 25:
> But she persisted and cried bitterly, a cry that would arouse pity. 'Please help me'.

Verse 26:
> He answered: 'It is not fair to give to you people what is meant for our own people'.

It is common knowledge that immigrants are looked down upon. They were often accused of being thieves. They have to get by with whatever is available, so she did not argue?

Verse 27:
> She responded with great humility: 'Yes what you say is true. It is not right to take what is meant for your people and give it to us, but even we need to survive, and right now it is the health of my only child'.

Verse 28:
> Then he said to her: 'You have moved me, come into the house so that I can look at the child.' And the woman went with him into the house.

Song
The leader may choose any appropriate song.

Closing Prayer
The Lord's Prayer

By Cheryl Dibeela

5. Age Based Discrimination

DISCRIMINATION OF CHILDREN
Sermon Text: Mark 10:13-16

Instructions: Get children to do a sketch of a scene where children are desperately trying to get to Jesus, but older people are preventing them.

Introduction

The HIV/AIDS pandemic has impacted negatively on the well-being of children in Africa. As parents and guardians have died, the number of orphans, vulnerable children and child-headed households has increased. The reality of parent to child transmission has also meant that some children are born HIV positive. While childhood used to be a period of much vitality and laughter, this is sadly no longer true for many children in Africa.

Age based discrimination should be a key theme for the church in Africa. The girl child in particular, faces the threat of rape as some infected male adults believe that sex with a virgin can revitalize them. Economic exploitation, the stigma of being labeled AIDS orphans, trauma and other factors weigh heavily on the children of Africa. The challenge for the church is how to allow children to accept Jesus' open invitation to them in the era of HIV/AIDS.

We Listen to the Word of God

The text shows how adults prevent children from associating with Jesus. While his disciples regard children as a nuisance, Jesus is quite open and welcoming towards the little ones. The children in the story are keen to have an encounter with Jesus and are inquisitive. In the context of HIV/AIDS, this need for faith and information is of utmost importance. There is also need to explore the question of how our societies could welcome children in the manner that Jesus did. Their forgiving quality is also important in dealing with HIV/AIDS issues.

We Apply the Word of God to Ourselves

WHAT CAN WE LEARN?
- Children require knowledge in HIV/AIDS contexts;
- Age-based discrimination should be resisted;
- Jesus welcomes children with open arms;
- HIV/AIDS threatens the well being of children; for example child-headed households;
- Adults need to be transformed and become like children, sincere and innocent, if they are to attain abundant life.

WHAT DO WE HAVE TO CONFESS?
- Sexual abuse of children in our families;
- Silence and misinformation surrounding children;
- Endangering children in child marriages;

- Abandoning care of children entirely to hired help;
- Exposing children through parent to child transmission of HIV.

WHAT CAN WE BE THANKFUL FOR?
- Churches and organizations that promote the welfare of children;
- That children continue to forgive and embrace despite their abuse;
- The gift of children;
- Churches that run day care centers, feeding and counseling centers.

WHAT CAN WE PRAY FOR?
- The suffering of children to be eliminated;
- For orphans and vulnerable children to receive education;
- That people would give generously towards the support of children;
- That the church would take children's ministry seriously.

We Apply the Word of God to the Congregation

Let children have the platform to express their fears and concerns in an era of HIV/AIDS.

Conclusion: A Word on Society

Governments should enact and enforce laws that protect the rights of children. The church and the media have an important role in disseminating information concerning HIV/AIDS to children. In addition, child sexual rape, pornography and other harmful trends should be severely punished. Society ought to become more child friendly so that children can enjoy their formative years.

Song
Any local chorus that celebrates children.
"We Are the World," (USA for Africa, 1986)

Prayer

Our Lord and Savior, Jesus Christ,
We commend the little ones to you.
You love them.
You shed your blood for them.
You taught us to value them.
Give us wisdom as we bring them up.
Let them grow into your faithful servants.
Abolish systems that choke them.
Heal their hurts.
Bring laughter into their joyful hearts.
Forgive us for denying them attention.
Empower us to recognize their significance.
In your precious name we pray. Amen

Suggested Objects/symbols/ideas: Doves; a painting of Jesus surrounded by children and playing with them, drawings by children, dolls, toys, a cradle, cloth used to tie a baby on its mother's back.
                                                                    By Ezra Chitando

DISCRIMINATION OF THE ELDERLY
Sermon Text: Genesis 18:1-15

Call to Prayer
Proverbs 4:5 –9

Get wisdom, get understanding,
Do not forget my words or swerve from them.
Do not forsake wisdom, and she will protect you;
Love her, and she will watch over you,
Wisdom is supreme; therefore get wisdom.
Though it cost all you have, get understanding.
Esteem her, and she will exalt you;
Embrace her, and she will honour you.
She will set a garland of grace on your head,
And present you with a crown of splendour.

Song (Chichewa)

Leader:	Ndinutu
All:	Ndinutu olemekezeka // (You are worthy of praise)
Leader:	Ndinutu
All:	Ndinutu opambana // (You are victorious)
Leader:	Nthawizonse // (All the time)
All:	Thawizonse simudzatisiya // (All the time you will never leave us or forsake us)
	Ndinutu opambana // (You are victorious)

	Leader: Ena // (Some)
All:	Ena atama magaleta // (Some trust in chariots)
Leader:	Ena // (Some)
All:	Ena akavalo // (Some in horses)
Leader:	Koma ine // (But me)
All:	Koma ine ndidzatama dzina // (But I will praise the name)
	Layehova mulungu wanga // (Of Jehovah my God)

(A Popular Malawian Chorus)

Introduction

There is an African proverb which says that with age comes wisdom. This proverb encourages the community to treat elderly people with respect, because of their wisdom accumulated over years through experience. However, in the era of HIV/AIDS, there are a lot of assumptions that are wrong and lead to the discrimination of old people in many ways. It is assumed that old people are responsible for taking care of their children when they have AIDS. Yet they do not get information about HIV/AIDS. They take on the responsibility of caregivers without the financial backing or physical strength to take care of the sick or orphans. As a result they get infected with HIV/AIDS through care giving. Most of the African cultural practices and beliefs assume that once women have reached menopause, they are no longer sexually active. Such assumptions discriminate against elderly people. What does God say about the sexual activities and right of elderly people?

We Listen to the Word of God

The leader or any member of the congregation can read Genesis 18 1-15. This passage can also be dramatized.

This passage is about the visit of three angelic beings to Abraham's' house, the hospitality of Abraham to the visitors, and the promise that Abraham's wife Sarah was going to have a baby boy.

DETAILS OF THE TEXT
➢ Three men visited Abraham. He identified one of them as the Lord. The other two must have been angelic beings. Abraham considered himself a servant of the visitors.

➢ Abraham begged the three men to stay and share a meal. He felt honored when they accepted his invitation. He then treated the visitors to Middle Eastern hospitality and food, which was his tradition.

➢ The message of the angels was that Sarah was going to have a son even through she had reached menopause, because nothing is too difficult for the Lord.

➢ Sarah found their message difficult to believe because of her age. But she is reminded that nothing is too difficult for the Lord.

We Apply the Word of God to Ourselves

WHAT CAN WE LEARN?
- That the Lord does not discriminate against elderly people. Although child birth is associated with young people, God is able to disregard biological rules and cause Sarah to have the pleasure of giving birth to a child;
- In order for Abraham and Sarah to have a child in their old age, God expected them to still have and enjoy their sexual relationship;
- God expects us to believe God's word and act on faith;
- That God keeps promises regardless natural laws;
- That the elderly people do have a sexual life.

WHAT DO WE HAVE TO CONFESS?
- We have allowed our cultural beliefs and practices to deny elderly people sexual pleasure;
- We have operated on wrong assumptions and denied elderly people information about HIV/AIDS;
- We have expected elderly people to be care givers for AIDS patients and orphans without supporting them with resources;
- We have exposed elderly people to the danger of contracting HIV by not equipping them with information and yet expect them to be primary caregivers.

WHAT CAN WE PRAY FOR?
- Forgiveness for abusing elderly people through our actions of discrimination;
- The protection of elderly people from HIV infection;
- Financial support for elderly people who are nursing the HIV infected patients and orphans;
- Strength and good health for elderly people as they look after AIDS patients and orphans.

We Apply the Word of God to the Congregation

WHAT CAN WE FEEL?
- Ashamed for abusing elderly people, who are our own parents and grand parents;
- Repentant for not giving elderly people information about HIV/AIDS, and thereby contributed towards their death through AIDS and stress;
- Sad that we have contributed towards denying elderly people sexual pleasure with their spouses.

WHAT CAN WE BE?
- A supporting community for elderly people;
- A teaching community to elderly people about HIV/AIDS;
- A caring community for elderly people; by organizing activities that dispel loneliness and promote community;
- Give support to grand parents caring for orphans.

WHAT CAN WE DO?
- Organize HIV/AIDS lessons for elderly people;
- Give elderly people the opportunities to acquire skills for entrepreneurship so that they can still be financially provided for in their old age;
- Organize seminars that affirm the celebration of sexuality among elderly couples;
- Involve elderly people in church activities;
- Provide relief for elderly people who are caregivers of AIDS patients and orphans, by giving them church raised love offerings.

Conclusion: A Word of God for Society

In our society today, we have the sick people, those suffering from HIV/AIDS and elderly people, whom we unfortunately discriminate against, even in the church. This discrimination against elderly people is ungodly and must not be practiced by Christians. It grieves God's heart. The elderly need to be given information about HIV/AIDS. Their sexuality needs to be affirmed as right and acceptable before God. Since they are responsible for taking care of the AIDS patients and orphans, they still need financial support from other members of the extended family, the church and the state.

Prayers

Leader:	Forgive us Lord, for ignoring the needs of elderly people.
All:	In your mercy, Lord, hear our prayer,
Leader:	Give us wisdom to plan how best to help elderly people who are overburdened with care giving of AIDS patients and orphans.
ALL:	In your mercy, Lord, hear our prayer

Song
The leader can choose a relevant song.

Benediction
May the Lord keep all of us until all our hairs are grey and until we walk with a third leg.

Symbols/objects/ideas: Testimonies of elderly people about care giving to AIDS and orphans, and traditional storytelling.

By Isabel Apawo Phiri

6. National Injustice

NATIONAL CORRUPTION
Sermon Text Luke 4:16-22

Introduction

The continent of Africa is rich in primary resources. However, looting by some African leaders and their partners abroad has resulted in the continent becoming hopelessly poor. National corruption undermines efforts to fight HIV/AIDS, as valuable resources are lost through such processes. Furthermore, national corruption results in the neglect of the poor, who are most vulnerable to HIV infection. Health and educational services suffer much neglect at the hands of corrupt and selfish leaders.

The church has an important prophetic role in the era of HIV/AIDS. It should be at the front line in demanding that African governments channel resources towards health services and the acquisition of drugs. In many African countries, funds are used in the construction of status symbols such as unnecessary expensive airports or soccer fields, ahead of more pressing issues in the area of health. In its preferential option for the poor, the church should be seen marching shoulder to shoulder with the infected and affected against national and international corruption.

We Listen to the Word of God

The passage is very clear that God is on the side of the oppressed. In the context of HIV/AIDS, these are the most vulnerable members of society. HIV/AIDS thrives in situations of poverty, and Christ declares that HIV/AIDS is an oppressive force. Furthermore, the passage proclaims freedom to those who heave under stifling systems. Women, children, displaced persons, prisoners and others who are most vulnerable to HIV/AIDS, should be empowered by this text.

We Apply the Word of God to Ourselves

WHAT CAN WE LEARN?
- HIV/AIDS is oppressive and should be tackled with passion;
- People living with HIV/AIDS (PLWHAs) require solidarity;
- The church should fight national corruption so that more people can access medical attention;
- That the healing is God's will for all;
- That Jesus took a stand against all forms of oppression.

WHAT DO WE HAVE TO CONFESS?
- Failure to fulfill the prophetic role in HIV/AIDS contexts;
- Being co-opted by the ruling elite;
- Being paralyzed by fear and frustration.

WHAT CAN WE BE THANKFUL FOR?
- That some church leaders have fought for the rights of PLWHA's;
- That some government leaders have resisted national corruption;
- The citizens who demand good governance and the observance of the rule of law;
- That the gospel gives the church a mandate to fight injustice.

WHAT CAN WE PRAY FOR?
- Courage to fight national and international corruption;
- Prophetic vision to support PLWHA's and fight injustice;
- Church efforts to identify with the poor.

We Apply the Word of God to the Congregation

Use a participatory session dealing with the following issues:
- Why does the church often simply look on when national resources are being looted?
- What are some of the pressing needs of PLWHAs?
- What is the church doing to support the vulnerable?
- What is the church to ensure that healing is for all?

Conclusion: A Word on Society

Leaders of organizations leading the fight against HIV/AIDS have sometimes been implicated in the embezzlement of funds meant for PLWHA's. In some instances, flashy cars have been bought, instead of supporting orphans and vulnerable children. It is important that leaders resist corrupt tendencies if the fight against the disease is to be won. Commitment towards the poor and disadvantaged members of society should guide all those who are central to this struggle. Above all, we should ask ourselves how HIV/AIDS resources can be brought to directly benefit the infected and affected rather than a few individuals running NGO's, etc.

Song

Ndasunungurwa tenda Ishe (2x)
Ndakanga ndakasungwa nemasimba aSatani
Ndasunungurwa tenda Ishe

I have been freed
Praise the Lord (2x)
I had been held captive by the devil's powers
I have been delivered, praise the Lord (2x)
(Popular chorus)

Prayer

God of liberation and justice,
Defender of the poor and marginalized,
We seek your guidance.
Give us the vision and confidence,
To become prophets when resources are looted.
Let us hear the cry of the widows.
Let us feed the orphans.
Let us denounce injustice by the powerful.
May we demand drugs for the sick.
May we demand care for the abandoned.
May we denounce wastefulness by the affluent.
Forgive our silence.
Forgive our complicity.
In your mercy, forgive our condemnation of PLWHA's
Forgive us when we deal lightly with the wounds of your people.
Forgive the times when we have offered artificial solutions.
Empower us to tackle corrupt systems.
Make us instruments of your peace.
Make us agents of transformation.
In Jesus' name we pray. Amen

Suggested Objects/symbols: Sackcloth (message of judgment), blood-dripping cloths (indicating the blood of the poor); wooden cross (Christ paid the price of suffering already), setting on the ashes, (to signify mourning and protest), newspapers that highlight the abuse of public funds.

By Ezra Chitando

7. International Injustice

INTERNATIONAL INJUSTICE
Sermon Text: Exodus 3:1-12

Introduction

At the beginning of the 21st century an international movement called the Jubilee movement came into being. This movement was a coalition of different groups such as the World Council of Churches, Oxfam, Christian Aid, and many others. This movement sought to address the question of international injustice that exists between countries in the north and those in the so-called 'third world'. Much of this international injustice exists because of the policies of global creditors such as the International Monetary Fund and the World Bank.

The jubilee movement still exists and continues with its mission, which is to call for the forgiveness of debts owed by 'Third World' countries to Western economies. This vision of a just world is important for the fight against HIV/AIDS. It is the poor who are most vulnerable to HIV/AIDS; they do not have all the information about the epidemic, they do not have the necessary access to antiretroviral drugs, they do not have access to testing programs, and they do not have enough food.

We Listen to the Word of God

DETAILS OF THE TEXT
This is one of the most important 'lessons' within the Torah or the Jewish law, which every boy and girl had to learn as part of their up bringing. The narrative was a source for prophetic preaching and it also featured a lot in cultic events.

In the narrative there are two characters; God and Moses. They are having a conversation, the subject of which is the plight of the Israelites/Hebrews in Egypt. The conversation is quite interesting and it might help for the worship leader to create dialogue between Moses and God and actually dramatize it (*see below*).

We Apply the Word of God to Ourselves and the Congregation

In this narrative God is decidedly interested in the plight of the Hebrew slaves in Egypt and wants to rescue them. God identifies a person to be the human agent of the rescue mission (liberation act). And the scene is now set for the greatest act of divine and human partnership in the liberation process.

WHAT DO WE LEARN?
God continues to be interested in the plight of the people of the world who suffer injustices. Most of these people are in the 'Third World', and they suffer at the hands of globalization and the elite in the West. Many of these people are denied affordable Anti-retroviral drugs to delay

their death from AIDS, they suffer from being used as cheap labour, and are watching the degradation of their environment. Despite these, God says 'I have seen the misery of my people,' and invites human agents to partner with God to release them.

WHAT CAN WE CONFESS?
We confess that:
- We do not, as churches, always take the side of the oppressed in our countries;
- Churches are often not vocal against international injustice;
- We often spiritualize the Bible, and as result miss out on its message that challenges political structures and institutions.

WHAT CAN WE BE THANKFUL FOR?
We thank God for:
- Those within and without the Church who fight for economic justice;
- For the New Partnership for Africa's Development (NEPAD), and the hope that it holds for Africa;
- For the spirit of renaissance in Africa;
- For the African Union and regional economic blocks;
- For the jubilee movement and what it seeks to achieve.

WHAT CAN WE PRAY FOR?
Let us pray:
- Liberator God we acknowledge your majesty.

You are Lord of the Church and the World

We pray that your justice become known to us,
May your people who live under the yoke of oppression
Experience relief and jubilee in their lives,
We pray for those who suffer from the burden of debt,
May they come to enjoy freedom from its clutches.
Amen

Suggested idea: Dramatic retelling
As Moses approaches the burning bush

God:	Moses, Moses!
Moses:	(*Startled*): Ye ....s! Who is there?
God:	It's me.
Moses:	Who?
God:	It's me, God.
Moses:	(*Puzzled*): God .... eh .... Which God?
God:	I am the God of your ancestors; the God Abraham, the God of Isaac, the God of Jacob, the God Mandela, Khama, the God of the women and children of Africa who suffer from AIDS.
Moses:	(*Afraid*) My goodness gracious! Lord have mercy!
God:	Moses, you are standing on holy ground. If I were you I would take off my shoes!

Moses takes off his sandals trembling and kneels down.

God: Moses, I have seen the misery of my people in Africa. I have heard them crying because of their taskmasters. Their suffering has greatly concerned me. So I have come to rescue them and to change their land so that it is no longer a land of oppression. So I want to you to go to the World Bank, the IMF, America and Europe and tell them to let my people go.

Moses: God!

God: Yes Moses

Moses: I mean … Well …Who am I really, to go to these bodies and tell them such news?

God: Don't worry Moses. It's not like I'll leave it all to you. I'll be there with you.

Song

We shall overcome, we shall overcome,
We shall overcome someday;
Oh deep in my heart I do believe,
We shall overcome some day.

We'll walk hand in hand….
The truth will make us free…
The Lord will see us through…
We shall live in peace…
We shall overcome….

(© Negro Spiritual)

By Moiseraele P. Dibeela

Selected Bibliography

Brienen, Francis ed. *"What does the Lord require?" A New Anthology of Prayers and Songs for Worship and Mission.* Norwich, Canterbury Press, 2000.

Byamugisha, Gideon; Steinitz, Lucy Y.; Williams, Glen; and Phumzile, Zondi. "Journey of Faith: Church-based Responses to HIV and AIDS in Three Southern African Countries". TALC, United Kingdom, 2002.

Donovan, Turner; and Hudson, Mary Lin. "Saved From Silence: Finding Women's Voice in Preaching". St Louis: Chalice Press, 1999.

Dube, Musa W. "Preaching to the Converted: Unsettling the Christian Church". *Ministerial Formation*, 93 (2001): 38-50.

_____. "Theological Challenges: Proclaiming the Fullness of Life in the HIV/AIDS and Global Economic Era". *International Review of Mission*, Vol. XCI/363, (2002): 535-549.

Dube, Musa W.; and Maluleke, Tinyiko S., eds. *Missionalia 29,* Special issue on HIV/AIDS and Theological Education, August, 2001.

Harling, Per, ed. "Worshipping Ecumenically: Orders of Service from Global Meetings with Suggestions for Local Use". *WCC Publications*, Geneva, 1995.

Isaack, Paul. "Health and Healing as a Challenge to Christian Ethics and Diaconal Ministry of the Church". *Black Theology: An International Journal*, Volume 2, (May 2003): 161-173.
.

Krieser, Matthias. "The Preacher's Helper: Sermon Preparations for Lutheran Lay Preachers". *Lutheran Church in Southern Africa*, Kanye, 2000.

Maluleke, Tinkyiko S. "Bible Study: The Graveyard Man, the Escaped Convict, and the Girl Child: A Mission of Awakening and Awakening of Mission". *International Review of Mission*, Vol. XCI/363, (2002): 550-557.

Maluleke, Tinyiko S.; and Nadar, Sarojini, eds. "Special Issue: Overcoming Violence against Women and Children". *Journal of Theology for Southern Africa,* Volume 114, 2002.

Olford, Stephen P. "Special-Day Sermon Outlines". *Grand Rapids: Bakers Books House Co.,*1997.

Karecke, Madge. "The Liturgy, Home of the Bible and Mission: First Steps in Rediscovering Their Relationship". (2000): 113-125.

Okure, Teresa, eds. "To Cast Fire Upon the Earth: Bible and Mission Collaborating in Today's Multicultural Global Context". *Cluster Publications*, Pietermaritzburg, 2000.

Trautwein, Dieter, eds. "Thuma Mina: International Ecumenical Hymnbook". Munchen-Berlin*, Basel Mission*, Berlin, 1995.

WCC. "Facing AIDS: The Challenge, the Churches' Response". *World Council of Churches*, Geneva, 1996.